DIABETES FACTS

50 QUESTIONS ABOUT DIABETES ANSWERED!

(SIMPLIFIED)

By

Dr. Chris Allan

Table of Contents

Dr. Chris Allan

INTRODUCTION

Welcome to the world of Diabetes Facts. This book is designed to take you on an exciting journey through the complicated and often misunderstood world of diabetes. The purpose of this book is to educate, enlighten, and inspire you with the latest information on diabetes, its causes, symptoms, and treatments.

Diabetes is a complex disease that affects millions of people worldwide, yet it is often misunderstood and shrouded in myths and misconceptions. This book aims to clear up those misconceptions and provide you with the facts about diabetes, from its earliest origins to the latest treatments.

The disease has been around for thousands of years, and has been described in ancient texts as "the sweet urine disease." However, it wasn't until the 20th century that scientists began to understand the complexities of diabetes and its impact on the human body.

Diabetes is a chronic disease that affects the way your body processes glucose (sugar). Glucose is the primary source of energy for your body's cells, but to be used by your cells, it needs to be converted into energy with the help of insulin. Insulin is a hormone produced by the pancreas that allows glucose to enter the cells and be used for energy.

When the body doesn't produce enough insulin or doesn't use it effectively, glucose accumulates in the bloodstream and can cause serious health problems. This is what happens in people with diabetes, where glucose builds up in their bloodstream instead of being absorbed by the cells, leading to high blood sugar levels.

There are two main types of diabetes: type 1 and type 2. Type 1 diabetes is an autoimmune disease where the body's immune system attacks and destroys the cells in the pancreas that produce insulin. Type 2 diabetes, on the other hand, is a metabolic disorder where the body becomes resistant to insulin or doesn't produce enough insulin to maintain normal blood sugar levels.

Diabetes affects people of all ages, races, and backgrounds. It can lead to serious complications, such as heart disease, kidney failure, blindness, and nerve damage. However, with proper management, people with diabetes can live healthy and fulfilling lives.

In this book, we will explore the latest research on diabetes, including its causes, risk factors, symptoms, and treatments. We will also discuss the different types of diabetes and the various complications that can arise from the disease. Additionally, we will explore the latest technological advances in diabetes management, such as insulin pumps and continuous glucose monitors.

We will also delve into the myths and misconceptions surrounding diabetes, such as whether it can be cured, and whether it's caused by eating too much sugar. We will examine the role of diet and exercise in diabetes management, and discuss the benefits of a healthy lifestyle in preventing and managing diabetes.

Finally, we will share interesting facts about diabetes. These facts will arm you with information at your fingertips, diabetes does not have to be a barrier to living a fulfilling life.

In conclusion, this book is designed to be a comprehensive guide to diabetes, providing you with the latest information and research on this complex disease.

Whether you are living with diabetes or know someone who is, this book will provide you with the knowledge and inspiration to take control of your health and live your best life. With the right knowledge, the right connections you have little or nothing to worry. This question and answer book for diabetes covers all you need to know and in the course of my profession I have come to know and believe that the quickest way to learn is to ask questions, get the answers and act on them, the knowledge stays with you a lifetime. So, buckle up and get ready for an exciting journey into the world of diabetes facts.

SECTION 1

KNOW ABOUT DIABETES

1. What is diabetes and how does it affect the body?

Diabetes is a chronic medical condition characterized by high levels of sugar (glucose) in the blood. It occurs when the body can't properly use or produce insulin, a hormone that regulates blood sugar levels.

Type 1 diabetes is an autoimmune disease where the immune system destroys insulin-producing cells in the pancreas, while type 2 diabetes is caused by insulin resistance, where cells don't respond effectively to insulin. High blood sugar levels can damage various organs and tissues, including the eyes, kidneys, nerves, and blood vessels. Over time, this can lead to serious health problems such as blindness, kidney failure, nerve damage, heart disease, and stroke.

Symptoms of diabetes may include increased thirst and hunger, frequent urination, fatigue, blurred vision, and slow wound healing. Treatment typically involves lifestyle modifications, such as diet and exercise, as well as medications and insulin therapy for type 1 diabetes. Early diagnosis and proper management are essential to prevent complications and improve quality of life for people with diabetes.

2. What are the different types of diabetes, and how do they differ ?

There are three main types of diabetes: Type 1, Type 2, and gestational diabetes.

Type 1 diabetes is an autoimmune disease in which the immune system attacks and destroys the insulin-producing cells in the pancreas. As a result, the body is unable to produce insulin, a hormone that regulates blood sugar levels. Type 1 diabetes is typically diagnosed in childhood or early adulthood, and requires daily insulin injections to manage blood sugar levels.

Type 2 diabetes is the most common form of diabetes, accounting for around 90% of all cases. In Type 2 diabetes, the body becomes resistant to insulin, and the pancreas may also gradually lose its ability to produce insulin. This can be caused by a combination of genetic and lifestyle factors, such as obesity and a lack of physical activity. Type 2 diabetes can often be managed through lifestyle changes, such as a healthy diet and regular exercise, as well as medications and insulin injections if necessary.

Gestational diabetes occurs during pregnancy and typically resolves after the baby is born. It occurs when the body is unable to produce enough insulin to regulate blood sugar levels during pregnancy, leading to high blood sugar levels. Gestational diabetes can increase the risk of complications during pregnancy and delivery, as well as the risk of Type 2 diabetes later in life.

Other less common types of diabetes include monogenic diabetes, which is caused by mutations in a single gene, and cystic fibrosis-related diabetes, which occurs in people with cystic fibrosis.

3. What are the common symptoms of diabetes, and how can they be managed ?

There are two main types of diabetes: type 1 and type 2. The common symptoms of diabetes include:

Increased thirst: People with diabetes often experience an unquenchable thirst due to the excess sugar in their bloodstream. As a result, they may drink more fluids than usual.

Frequent urination: Diabetes can cause the kidneys to work harder to filter the excess sugar from the bloodstream, resulting in increased urine production.

Fatigue: Because the body is unable to use glucose effectively, people with diabetes may feel tired and weak, even if they have not exerted themselves.

Weight loss: In type 1 diabetes, the body is unable to produce insulin, which can lead to rapid weight loss. In type 2 diabetes, weight loss may occur due to increased urination and a decrease in appetite.

Slow healing of wounds: High blood sugar levels can damage the blood vessels and nerves, which can cause wounds to heal slowly.

Blurred vision: High blood sugar levels can also cause changes in the shape of the lens of the eye, leading to blurred vision.

Numbness and tingling in the hands and feet: High blood sugar levels can damage the nerves, causing numbness and tingling in the hands and feet.

4. What are the risk factors for developing diabetes?

There are several risk factors that increase the likelihood of developing diabetes. We will discuss some of the most common risk factors for diabetes.

Age: The risk of developing diabetes increases as people get older. This is because aging is associated with decreased physical activity, decreased muscle mass, and increased body fat, all of which can contribute to insulin resistance and high blood sugar levels.

Family history: Diabetes tends to run in families, and having a close relative with diabetes increases the risk of developing the disease. This is thought to be due to a combination of genetic and environmental factors.

Obesity: Being overweight or obese is a major risk factor for diabetes. Excess body fat can make it harder for the body to use insulin effectively, leading to insulin resistance and high blood sugar levels.

Physical inactivity: Lack of physical activity can also contribute to insulin resistance and high blood sugar levels. Regular exercise helps the body use insulin more effectively and can help prevent or manage diabetes.

Gestational diabetes: Women who develop gestational diabetes during pregnancy are at increased risk of developing type 2 diabetes later in life.

High blood pressure: High blood pressure can damage the blood vessels and increase the risk of developing diabetes. People with high blood pressure should monitor their blood sugar levels and work with their healthcare provider to manage their risk for diabetes.

High cholesterol: High levels of LDL (bad) cholesterol and low levels of HDL (good) cholesterol are associated with an increased risk of developing diabetes.

Smoking: Smoking increases the risk of developing diabetes, as well as other serious health problems such as heart disease and lung cancer.

Ethnicity: Certain ethnic groups, such as African Americans, Hispanic/Latino Americans, Native

Americans, and Asian Americans, are at higher risk of developing diabetes.

Polycystic ovary syndrome (PCOS): PCOS is a hormonal disorder that affects women of reproductive age. Women with PCOS are at increased risk of developing insulin resistance and diabetes.

5. How does a family history of diabetes affect your risk of developing the disease?

A family history of diabetes can significantly increase an individual's risk of developing the disease. There are two types of diabetes: type 1 and type 2. Type 1 diabetes is an autoimmune disorder that usually affects children and young adults, while type 2 diabetes is a metabolic disorder that can develop at any age and is typically associated with lifestyle factors such as poor diet and lack of physical activity.

Type 1 Diabetes:

Family history plays a significant role in the development of type 1 diabetes. According to the American Diabetes Association (ADA), if a parent has type 1 diabetes, a child has a 6% chance of developing the condition. If both parents have type 1 diabetes, the risk increases to 30%. In contrast, the general population has a 0.4% risk of developing type 1 diabetes.

Type 1 diabetes is caused by a combination of genetic and environmental factors. Specific genes are responsible for the development of type 1 diabetes, and research has identified more than 50 genes associated with the disease. However, having these genes does not guarantee that an individual will develop type 1 diabetes. Environmental factors such as viral infections, exposure to toxins, and diet can trigger the disease in those with a genetic predisposition.

Type 2 Diabetes:

Family history is also a significant risk factor for type 2 diabetes. According to the ADA, if a parent or sibling has type 2 diabetes, an individual's risk of developing the condition increases by two to three times. If both parents have type 2 diabetes, the risk increases up to six times.

Type 2 diabetes is brought on by a combination of genetic and environmental factors, just like type 1 diabetes. An individual's risk of developing type 2 diabetes is significantly influenced by genetics. Over 400 genes have been linked to the condition, according to the research. These qualities can influence how the body processes glucose, insulin, and different chemicals that manage glucose levels.

However, other aspects of one's lifestyle, such as a poor diet and inactivity, are also significant contributors to the onset of type 2 diabetes. A sedentary lifestyle can raise an individual's risk of obesity, which is a major risk factor for type 2 diabetes. Type 2 diabetes can also be brought on by a poor diet, especially one that is high in sugar and refined carbohydrates.

6. Can obesity cause diabetes, and if so, how?

Obesity is a significant risk factor for developing diabetes. Its is a condition where a person has excess body fat. Obesity is generally defined by body mass index (BMI), a ratio of weight to height. A BMI of 30 or higher is considered obese. Obesity is associated with many health problems, including cardiovascular disease, hypertension, sleep apnea, and type 2 diabetes.

Obesity contributes to the development of type 2 diabetes in several ways. One of the primary mechanisms is through insulin resistance. Insulin resistance is a condition where the body's cells become less responsive to insulin, making it more difficult for glucose to enter the cells. As a result, glucose accumulates in the bloodstream, leading to high blood sugar levels. Obesity increases the risk of insulin resistance, which can eventually lead to the development of type 2 diabetes.

Another way that obesity contributes to the development of type 2 diabetes is through inflammation. Obesity is associated with chronic low-grade inflammation, which can damage the body's cells and tissues. This inflammation can impair insulin signaling and lead to insulin resistance. Additionally, obesity can contribute to the dysfunction of the beta cells in the pancreas, which produce insulin. Over time, the beta cells may become exhausted and fail to produce enough insulin, leading to high blood sugar levels.

Finally, obesity can contribute to the development of type 2 diabetes by altering the levels of hormones that regulate glucose metabolism. Adipose tissue (fat) produces several hormones that can impact glucose metabolism, including leptin, adiponectin, and resistin. Obesity can alter the levels of these hormones, leading to impaired glucose metabolism and increased risk of type 2 diabetes.

7. What role does insulin play in diabetes, and how does it affect the body?

Insulin is a hormone produced by the pancreas that plays a critical role in regulating blood glucose levels. Diabetes is a metabolic disorder characterized by high blood sugar levels due to the body's inability to produce or effectively use insulin. We will explore the role of insulin in diabetes and how it affects the body.

Insulin and Glucose Regulation

When we eat carbohydrates, they are broken down into glucose, which is absorbed into the bloodstream. As blood glucose levels rise, the pancreas produces insulin and releases it into the bloodstream. Insulin helps transport glucose from the bloodstream into cells throughout the body, where it can be used for energy. Insulin also signals the liver to store excess glucose as glycogen for future use.

Insulin Resistance and Type 2 Diabetes

In type 2 diabetes, the body becomes resistant to insulin, which means that cells are no longer able to effectively use insulin to transport glucose into the cells. As a result, blood glucose levels remain high, and the pancreas must produce more insulin to compensate. Over time, the pancreas may not be able to keep up with the demand for insulin, leading to high blood glucose levels and a diagnosis of diabetes.

Insulin and Type 1 Diabetes

In type 1 diabetes, the immune system attacks and destroys the cells in the pancreas that produce insulin. Without insulin, glucose cannot enter cells, and it builds up in the bloodstream, leading to high blood glucose levels. People with type 1 diabetes must take insulin injections or use an insulin pump to manage their blood glucose levels.

Effects of High Blood Glucose Levels

High blood glucose levels can have serious long-term effects on the body. Over time, high blood glucose levels can damage blood vessels and nerves, leading to complications such as:

Cardiovascular disease: High blood glucose levels can damage blood vessels, increasing the risk of heart attack, stroke, and other cardiovascular diseases.

Kidney disease: High blood glucose levels can damage the kidneys, leading to kidney disease.

Eye damage: High blood glucose levels can damage the blood vessels in the eyes, leading to diabetic retinopathy, which can cause vision loss.

Nerve damage: High blood glucose levels can damage the nerves, leading to diabetic neuropathy, which can cause numbness, tingling, and pain in the hands, feet, and legs.

Foot damage: High blood glucose levels can damage the blood vessels and nerves in the feet, leading to poor circulation, foot ulcers, and even amputation.

Effects of Low Blood Glucose Levels

Insulin plays a crucial role in preventing low blood glucose levels, or hypoglycemia. Hypoglycemia occurs when blood glucose levels drop too low, usually below 70 mg/dL. Common symptoms of hypoglycemia include:

Shakiness

Dizziness

Sweating

Hunger

Headache

Confusion

Irritability

Weakness

If left untreated, severe hypoglycemia can cause seizures, loss of consciousness, and even death. People with diabetes who take insulin must monitor their blood glucose levels closely and take steps to prevent hypoglycemia, such as eating regular meals and snacks, adjusting their insulin doses as needed, and carrying a source of glucose (such as candy or juice) with them at all times.

Insulin plays a critical role in regulating blood glucose levels, and diabetes occurs when the body is unable to produce or effectively use insulin.

8. How does the body regulate blood sugar levels, and what happens when this system is disrupted?

The regulation of blood sugar levels is a vital physiological process that is primarily controlled by two hormones: insulin and glucagon. These hormones work in tandem to maintain blood glucose levels within a specific range, typically between 70 and 100 mg/dL. When this system is disrupted, it can lead to a range of health problems, including diabetes and hypoglycemia.

Insulin is secreted by the beta cells of the pancreas in response to elevated blood glucose levels. When blood glucose levels rise, insulin is released into the bloodstream, where it acts to lower blood glucose levels by facilitating the uptake of glucose by cells. Insulin binds to insulin receptors on the surface of cells, allowing glucose to enter the cell and be used as energy or stored as glycogen.

Glucagon, on the other hand, is secreted by the alpha cells of the pancreas when blood glucose levels are low. Glucagon acts to raise blood glucose levels by stimulating the liver to convert stored glycogen into glucose, which is released into the bloodstream.

Together, insulin and glucagon work to maintain blood glucose homeostasis. In a healthy individual, blood glucose levels remain relatively stable, with insulin and glucagon working in a delicate balance to ensure that glucose is available to cells when needed.

When this system is disrupted, it can lead to a range of health problems. In diabetes, for example, the body is unable to produce or properly use insulin, leading to elevated blood glucose levels. Over time, this can lead to a range of complications, including nerve damage, kidney disease, and cardiovascular disease.

In hypoglycemia, on the other hand, blood glucose levels drop too low, which can cause symptoms such as dizziness, confusion, and even seizures. This can be caused by a range of factors, including medication side effects, excessive alcohol consumption, and certain medical conditions.

Another condition that can disrupt blood sugar regulation is insulin resistance. In this condition, the body produces insulin, but the cells become resistant to its effects, meaning that glucose cannot enter the cell as effectively. This can lead to elevated blood glucose levels and is a precursor to type 2 diabetes.

The regulation of blood sugar levels is a complex physiological process that is primarily controlled by the hormones insulin and glucagon. When this system is disrupted, it can lead to a range of health problems, including diabetes, hypoglycemia, and insulin resistance.

9. Can stress or anxiety trigger diabetes, and if so, how?

Stress and anxiety can have a significant impact on our bodies, both physically and mentally. While they may not directly trigger diabetes, stress and anxiety can lead to changes in blood glucose levels and may increase the risk of developing type 2 diabetes over time.

When we experience stress or anxiety, our bodies release stress hormones such as cortisol and adrenaline. These hormones increase our heart rate, elevate blood pressure, and cause our bodies to release glucose from the liver. This glucose is intended to provide our muscles with energy to respond to the perceived threat. However, if we do not use the energy, the glucose can build up in our bloodstream, leading to high blood sugar levels.

Over time, repeated episodes of stress and anxiety can cause our bodies to become less sensitive to insulin, the hormone that regulates blood glucose levels. When our bodies become resistant to insulin, it can result in elevated blood glucose levels and a higher risk of developing type 2 diabetes.

In addition to its effect on blood glucose levels, stress and anxiety can also lead to unhealthy behaviors that increase the risk of diabetes. For example, when we feel stressed or anxious, we may be more likely to reach for unhealthy comfort foods or skip exercise, which can contribute to weight gain and increase the risk of type 2 diabetes.

It is important to note that stress and anxiety are not the sole causes of diabetes, and many other factors can contribute to its development, including genetics, lifestyle factors, and other medical conditions. However, managing stress and anxiety can be an important part of preventing and managing diabetes.

10. What is the link between diabetes and cardiovascular disease, and how can this risk be minimized?

Diabetes and cardiovascular disease (CVD) are closely related, with diabetes being a significant risk factor for the development of CVD. In fact, individuals with diabetes are two to four times more likely to develop CVD than those without diabetes. We will explore the link between diabetes and CVD, and discuss strategies to minimize the risk.

Diabetes is a chronic condition characterized by high blood glucose levels, resulting from the body's inability to produce or use insulin effectively. CVD is a term that encompasses a group of conditions that affect the heart and blood vessels, including coronary artery disease, heart failure, and stroke. People with diabetes are at an increased risk of developing these conditions due to several factors, including:

Elevated Blood Glucose Levels: High blood glucose levels can damage the lining of blood vessels, leading to the development of atherosclerosis, a condition in which plaque accumulates in the walls of arteries, restricting blood flow and increasing the risk of heart attack and stroke.

Dyslipidemia: Diabetes can lead to abnormal lipid profiles, with increased levels of triglycerides and decreased levels of high-density lipoprotein (HDL) cholesterol. This lipid profile is associated with an increased risk of atherosclerosis and CVD.

Hypertension: People with diabetes are more likely to have high blood pressure, which is a major risk factor for CVD.

Inflammation: Diabetes is associated with chronic low-grade inflammation, which can contribute to the development of atherosclerosis.

Obesity: Obesity is a risk factor for both diabetes and CVD. Excess body weight increases the risk of developing diabetes, and it also puts additional strain on the heart and blood vessels, increasing the risk of CVD.

To minimize the risk of CVD in individuals with diabetes, several strategies can be employed:

Glycemic Control: Maintaining optimal blood glucose levels is essential to prevent the development of complications associated with diabetes, including CVD.

Individuals with diabetes should aim to keep their HbA1c levels below 7%.

Blood Pressure Control: Blood pressure control is crucial in minimizing the risk of CVD in individuals with diabetes. The target blood pressure for people with diabetes is below 130/80 mmHg.

Lipid Management: Individuals with diabetes should have regular lipid profiles to monitor their cholesterol levels. The target levels for LDL cholesterol should be below 100 mg/dL, and HDL cholesterol levels should be above 40 mg/dL for men and above 50 mg/dL for women.

Lifestyle Modifications: Lifestyle modifications can help individuals with diabetes manage their blood glucose levels and minimize the risk of CVD. These modifications include maintaining a healthy weight, engaging in regular physical activity, avoiding smoking, and following a healthy diet that is low in saturated and trans fats and high in fruits, vegetables, and whole grains.

Medications: Several medications are available to minimize the risk of CVD in individuals with diabetes. These include aspirin, which can reduce the risk of heart attack and stroke, and statins, which can lower cholesterol levels and reduce the risk of CVD.

As a wrap, diabetes and CVD are closely related, with diabetes being a significant risk factor for the development of CVD. To minimize the risk of CVD in individuals with diabetes, it is essential to maintain optimal glycemic control, blood pressure control, and lipid management. Lifestyle modifications and medications can also help individuals with diabetes manage their blood glucose levels and minimize the risk of CVD.

11. Is there a link between diabetes and cancer, and if so, what is it?

Diabetes and cancer are two of the most prevalent health conditions worldwide. Both diseases affect millions of people every year, and research suggests that there may be a link between the two. This link is not fully understood, but scientists have identified several potential connections that are worth exploring. Here we will explore the link between diabetes and cancer, looking at the potential causes and the evidence supporting the connection.

First, let's define diabetes and cancer. Diabetes is a chronic metabolic disorder characterized by high blood glucose levels. This occurs because the body is unable to produce or use insulin, a hormone that helps to regulate blood sugar levels. Cancer, on the other hand, is a group of diseases characterized by the uncontrolled growth and spread of abnormal cells in the body.

Now, let's explore the potential links between diabetes and cancer. One possible connection is the role of insulin. Insulin helps to regulate blood sugar levels by signaling to cells to absorb glucose from the bloodstream. However, research has shown that insulin can also promote the growth of cancer cells. This is because cancer cells have insulin receptors on their surface, which allows them to absorb more glucose and use it for energy. This means that people with diabetes, who have higher insulin levels, may be at a higher risk of developing certain types of cancer, such as breast, colon, and pancreatic cancer.

Another potential link between diabetes and cancer is chronic inflammation. Diabetes is associated with chronic inflammation, which is a condition where the body's immune system is constantly activated. Chronic inflammation can damage cells and tissues in the body, increasing the risk of cancer. Inflammation is also a hallmark of cancer, as cancer cells release inflammatory molecules that can promote the growth and spread of tumors. This means that people with diabetes may be more susceptible to cancer due to the chronic inflammation associated with their condition.

Obesity is another potential link between diabetes and cancer. Obesity is a major risk factor for both diabetes and cancer, and research suggests that the two conditions may be linked. Obesity increases the risk of insulin resistance, which can lead to diabetes. It also promotes chronic inflammation and hormonal imbalances in the body, both of which can increase the risk of cancer. This means that people who are overweight or obese may be at a higher risk of developing both diabetes and cancer.

There is also evidence to suggest that certain diabetes medications may increase the risk of cancer. For example, some studies have shown that long-term use of metformin, a commonly prescribed diabetes medication, may increase the risk of pancreatic cancer. However, other studies have found no such association, and more research is needed to fully understand the relationship between diabetes medications and cancer.

So, what can be done to reduce the risk of cancer in people with diabetes? One approach is to manage diabetes through lifestyle changes and medication. This includes maintaining a healthy weight, exercising regularly, and following a balanced diet that is low in sugar and processed foods. These lifestyle changes can help to regulate blood sugar levels, reduce chronic inflammation, and lower the risk of cancer.

In conclusion, the link between diabetes and cancer is complex and multifaceted. Insulin resistance, chronic inflammation, obesity, and certain diabetes medications are all potential factors that may increase the risk of cancer in people with diabetes.

12. What are the long-term complications of diabetes, and how can they be prevented?

Diabetes is a chronic disease characterized by high levels of blood sugar (glucose) due to either insufficient insulin production or insulin resistance. Over time, diabetes can lead to serious health complications affecting various organs and systems in the body. The long-term complications of diabetes can be prevented or delayed by maintaining good blood glucose, blood pressure, and cholesterol control through healthy lifestyle habits and medications.

The long-term complications of diabetes can be divided into two categories: macrovascular and microvascular complications. Macrovascular complications refer to diseases of the large blood vessels that supply the heart, brain, and legs. Microvascular complications refer to diseases of the small blood vessels that supply the eyes, kidneys, and nerves.

Macrovascular complications include coronary artery disease, peripheral arterial disease, and stroke. People with diabetes have a higher risk of developing these conditions because high blood glucose levels can damage the lining of blood vessels, causing them to narrow and harden. This leads to a buildup of fatty deposits (plaque) that can block blood flow and cause a heart attack or stroke. Peripheral arterial disease occurs when the blood vessels that supply the legs and feet become narrowed or blocked, leading to pain, numbness, and poor wound healing. These complications can be prevented by controlling blood glucose levels, blood pressure, and cholesterol through a healthy diet, regular exercise, and medication.

Microvascular complications include diabetic retinopathy, nephropathy, and neuropathy. Diabetic retinopathy is a condition that affects the eyes and can lead to blindness. High blood glucose levels can damage the small blood vessels in the retina, causing them to leak or become blocked. This can lead to vision loss or blindness. Regular eye exams and good blood glucose control can prevent or delay the onset of diabetic retinopathy.

Diabetic nephropathy is a condition that affects the kidneys and can lead to kidney failure. High blood glucose levels can damage the small blood vessels in the kidneys, causing them to become leaky or blocked. This can lead to proteinuria (protein in the urine), high blood pressure, and kidney damage. Good blood glucose and blood pressure control, along with medications called angiotensin-converting enzyme inhibitors (ACE inhibitors) or angiotensin receptor blockers (ARBs), can prevent or delay the onset of diabetic nephropathy.

Diabetic neuropathy is a condition that affects the nerves and can lead to pain, numbness, and tingling in the hands and feet. High blood glucose levels can damage the small blood vessels that supply the nerves, leading to nerve damage. Good blood glucose control can prevent or delay the onset of diabetic neuropathy.

Other long-term complications of diabetes include skin conditions, such as bacterial and fungal infections, as well as hearing loss, depression, and cognitive decline. These complications can be prevented or delayed by controlling blood glucose levels, blood pressure, and cholesterol through a healthy lifestyle and medications.

Preventing or delaying the onset of the long-term complications of diabetes requires a multifaceted approach. A healthy diet that is low in saturated and trans fats, high in fiber, and rich in fruits, vegetables, and whole grains can help control blood glucose, blood pressure, and cholesterol. Regular physical activity, such as brisk walking, cycling, or swimming, can also help control blood glucose and blood pressure, as well as reduce the risk of heart disease and stroke.

In addition to lifestyle changes, medications are often necessary to control blood glucose, blood pressure, and cholesterol in people with diabetes. Oral medications, such as metformin, sulfonylureas, and thiazolidinediones can help.

13. What is the glycemic index, and how does it relate to diabetes?

The glycemic index (GI) is a measure of how quickly a carbohydrate-containing food raises blood sugar levels after consumption. The GI scale ranges from 0 to 100, with higher scores indicating that the food causes blood sugar levels to rise more quickly.

Foods with a high GI are rapidly broken down and absorbed by the body, leading to a sharp increase in blood sugar levels. This spike in blood sugar can be particularly problematic for people with diabetes, as their bodies either don't produce enough insulin (type 1 diabetes) or can't effectively use insulin (type 2 diabetes) to regulate blood sugar levels.

In contrast, foods with a low GI are digested and absorbed more slowly, leading to a more gradual increase in blood sugar levels. This gradual increase is less likely to cause blood sugar spikes and is therefore a better choice for people with diabetes.

While the GI is a useful tool for managing blood sugar levels, it is important to note that it is not the only factor to consider when making dietary choices. The amount and type of carbohydrates in a food, as well as the presence of other nutrients like protein and fiber, can also impact blood sugar levels.

It is also important to note that not all carbohydrates have the same impact on blood sugar levels. For example, complex carbohydrates, like those found in whole grains and legumes, are digested more slowly and have a lower GI than simple carbohydrates, like those found in sugary drinks and candy.

To use the GI to make dietary choices, individuals with diabetes can consult a GI chart or database to find the GI values of different foods. They can then aim to choose foods with a lower GI and pair them with protein and fiber to help slow the absorption of carbohydrates and prevent blood sugar spikes.

In addition to using the GI to make dietary choices, individuals with diabetes should also aim to maintain a healthy and balanced diet, engage in regular physical activity, and monitor their blood sugar levels regularly to help manage their condition.

The glycemic index is a useful tool for managing blood sugar levels in people with diabetes. By choosing foods with a lower GI and pairing them with protein and fiber, individuals with diabetes can help prevent blood sugar spikes and maintain healthy blood sugar levels. However, it is important to use the GI in conjunction with other dietary and lifestyle factors to effectively manage diabetes.

14. What are some common foods that can cause spikes in blood sugar levels?

Blood sugar, also known as blood glucose, is a vital source of energy for the body's cells. However, when blood sugar levels get too high, it can cause a range of health problems, including diabetes, obesity, and heart disease. Some foods can cause a rapid increase in blood sugar levels, which can be harmful to those with diabetes and those who are trying to manage their blood sugar levels. We will discuss some common foods that can cause spikes in blood sugar levels.

White bread, pasta, and rice:

White bread, pasta, and rice are all high in refined carbohydrates, which can cause a spike in blood sugar levels. These foods are quickly digested and absorbed by the body, leading to a rapid rise in blood sugar levels. Instead, it's better to choose whole grain bread, pasta, and brown rice, which contain fiber that slows down digestion and absorption, resulting in a slower and steadier increase in blood sugar levels.

Sugary drinks:

Sugary drinks such as soda, fruit juice, and energy drinks are high in sugar and can cause a rapid spike in blood sugar levels. These drinks provide empty calories and contribute to weight gain, which can increase the risk of developing diabetes and other health problems.

Candy and sweets:

Candy and sweets are high in sugar and can cause a rapid spike in blood sugar levels. These foods provide empty calories and contribute to weight gain, which can increase the risk of developing diabetes and other health problems. It's better to choose fruits or nuts as a snack instead.

French fries and potato chips:

French fries and potato chips are high in refined carbohydrates and can cause a rapid spike in blood sugar levels. These foods are also high in fat and calories, which can contribute to weight gain and increase the risk of developing diabetes and other health problems.

Processed meats:

Processed meats such as hot dogs, bacon, and sausage are high in fat and sodium and can cause a rapid spike in blood sugar levels. These foods are also associated with an increased risk of heart disease and cancer. Instead, it's better to choose lean proteins such as chicken, fish, and legumes.

High-fat dairy:

High-fat dairy products such as whole milk, cheese, and butter are high in saturated fat and can cause a rapid spike in blood sugar levels. These foods are also associated with an increased risk of heart disease and other health problems. Instead, it's better to choose low-fat or fat-free dairy products such as skim milk, low-fat cheese, and yogurt.

Alcohol:

Alcohol can cause a rapid spike in blood sugar levels, especially when consumed on an empty stomach. Drinking alcohol can also impair the body's ability to regulate blood sugar levels, which can be especially harmful for those with diabetes. It's better to limit alcohol consumption and choose low-sugar options such as wine or light beer.

Dried fruit:

Dried fruit is a concentrated source of sugar and can cause a rapid spike in blood sugar levels. While dried fruit does contain some nutrients and fiber, it's better to choose fresh fruits instead, which are lower in sugar and higher in water content.

Breakfast cereals:

Many breakfast cereals are high in sugar and refined carbohydrates and can cause a rapid spike in blood sugar levels. Instead, it's better to choose whole grain cereals that are low in sugar and high in fiber.

Smoothies:

Smoothies can be a healthy option, but many store-bought varieties are high in sugar and can cause a rapid spike in blood sugar levels. It's better to make your own smoothies with fresh or frozen fruits and vegetables and low-sugar options such as almond milk or plain yogurt.

15. How can a person with diabetes manage their diet to minimize the risk of complications?

For individuals with diabetes, managing their diet is crucial to minimize the risk of complications such as cardiovascular disease, nerve damage, and kidney disease.

Here are some practical and realistic suggestions to manage your diet and minimize the risk of complications:

Focus on whole foods:

Whole foods such as vegetables, fruits, whole grains, lean proteins, and healthy fats should be the cornerstone of a healthy diet for individuals with diabetes. These foods are nutrient-dense and contain fiber, which can help regulate blood sugar levels.

Limit processed foods:

Processed foods are often high in added sugars, unhealthy fats, and sodium, which can lead to weight gain, insulin resistance, and high blood pressure. Limit your intake of processed foods and try to make your meals from scratch using whole ingredients.

Eat regularly:

Eating regular meals and snacks throughout the day can help regulate blood sugar levels and prevent spikes and crashes. Aim to eat three meals and two to three snacks per day, spaced out evenly.

Monitor portion sizes:

Controlling portion sizes is essential for managing blood sugar levels and preventing weight gain. Use measuring cups or a food scale to portion out your meals and snacks, and try to eat slowly and mindfully.

Choose healthy carbohydrates:

Carbohydrates can have a significant impact on blood sugar levels, so it's crucial to choose healthy options. Focus on whole grains, such as brown rice, quinoa, and whole-wheat pasta, and avoid refined carbohydrates like white bread, white rice, and sugary drinks.

Limit added sugars:

Added sugars can cause blood sugar levels to spike and can lead to weight gain and other health problems. Try to limit your intake of added sugars and avoid sugary drinks, desserts, and processed foods.

Choose healthy fats:

Healthy fats, such as those found in nuts, seeds, avocado, and olive oil, can help improve blood sugar control and lower the risk of heart disease. Aim to include healthy fats in your meals and snacks.

Limit saturated and trans fats:

Saturated and trans fats can increase the risk of heart disease and should be limited in the diet. Avoid processed foods that are high in saturated and trans fats, and choose lean proteins such as chicken, fish, and tofu.

Drink plenty of water:

Drinking plenty of water can help regulate blood sugar levels, prevent dehydration, and aid in weight loss. Aim to drink at least eight cups of water per day.

Seek professional advice:

Consulting a registered dietitian who specializes in diabetes management can be an excellent resource for learning how to manage your diet effectively. A dietitian can help you create a personalized meal plan that meets your nutritional needs and fits your lifestyle.

16. What role do carbohydrates play in managing blood sugar levels for people with diabetes?

Carbohydrates are an essential nutrient for the body and serve as a primary source of energy. For people with diabetes, managing carbohydrate intake is essential in maintaining healthy blood sugar levels. When carbohydrates are consumed, they are broken down into glucose, which enters the bloodstream and causes blood sugar levels to rise. Therefore, controlling carbohydrate intake is crucial for managing diabetes.

Here are some practical and realistic suggestions for managing blood sugar levels through carbohydrate intake:

Monitor carbohydrate intake: It is crucial to monitor the amount and type of carbohydrates consumed. A registered dietitian can help create a personalized meal plan that includes the right balance of carbohydrates, protein, and fat. People with diabetes should aim to consume complex carbohydrates, such as whole grains, fruits, vegetables, and legumes, which have a lower glycemic index and are slower to digest, resulting in a slower and steadier rise in blood sugar levels.

Avoid simple carbohydrates: Simple carbohydrates, such as sugar and refined carbohydrates, are quickly digested and can cause a rapid spike in blood sugar levels. Therefore, it is recommended to limit or avoid foods and beverages containing added sugars, such as candy, soda, and processed snacks.

Consider portion sizes: Eating too much of any food, including carbohydrates, can cause blood sugar levels to rise. Therefore, it is important to monitor portion sizes and stick to recommended serving sizes.

Eat regularly: Eating meals and snacks regularly can help manage blood sugar levels by preventing significant fluctuations. People with diabetes should aim to eat small, frequent meals throughout the day rather than skipping meals or eating large meals.

Choose high-fiber foods: High-fiber foods, such as fruits, vegetables, whole grains, and legumes, can help slow down the absorption of carbohydrates, resulting in a slower rise in blood sugar levels. Aim to include at least five servings of fruits and vegetables per day and choose whole grains over refined grains.

Use the glycemic index: The glycemic index ranks foods based on how quickly they raise blood sugar levels. Foods with a higher glycemic index are digested more quickly, resulting in a more rapid increase in blood sugar levels. Using the glycemic index can help people with diabetes make informed choices about the types of carbohydrates they consume. Foods with a lower glycemic index, such as whole grains, fruits, and vegetables, are ideal choices.

Choose low-carbohydrate snacks: When snacking, it is important to choose low-carbohydrate options to prevent blood sugar levels from spiking. Good options include nuts, seeds, vegetables, and protein-rich snacks.

Consider carbohydrate counting: Carbohydrate counting is a method of tracking carbohydrate intake to help manage blood sugar levels. People with diabetes can work with a registered dietitian to determine the appropriate number of carbohydrates to consume each day and how to count carbohydrates.

Monitor blood sugar levels: Regular monitoring of blood sugar levels can help people with diabetes determine how different foods and activities affect their blood sugar levels. People with diabetes should aim to monitor their blood sugar levels regularly, as recommended by their healthcare provider.

Managing carbohydrate intake is essential for people with diabetes in maintaining healthy blood sugar levels. By monitoring carbohydrate intake, avoiding simple carbohydrates, considering portion sizes, eating regularly, choosing high-fiber foods, using the glycemic index, choosing low-carbohydrate snacks, considering carbohydrate counting, and monitoring blood sugar levels, people with diabetes can effectively manage their blood sugar levels and maintain good health. Working with a registered dietitian can help people with diabetes create a personalized meal plan that meets their individual needs and preferences.

17. Can certain types of fats or oils increase the risk of developing diabetes?

Yes, certain types of fats and oils can increase the risk of developing diabetes. The evidence supporting this claim comes from various studies conducted on the relationship between dietary fat intake and diabetes risk.

Diabetes is a metabolic disorder characterized by high blood sugar levels due to insulin resistance or deficiency. There are two main types of diabetes: type 1, which is an autoimmune disease that usually occurs in childhood or adolescence, and type 2, which is more common and is associated with lifestyle factors such as diet, physical inactivity, and obesity.

Type 2 diabetes accounts for about 90% of all cases and is largely preventable through lifestyle modifications such as maintaining a healthy weight, engaging in regular physical activity, and following a healthy diet.

One important aspect of a healthy diet is the type and amount of fat consumed. Dietary fats are essential for many bodily functions, such as providing energy, insulating and protecting organs, and aiding in the absorption of fat-soluble vitamins. However, excessive intake of certain types of fats can have detrimental effects on health, including an increased risk of developing type 2 diabetes.

Saturated fats, which are solid at room temperature and mainly found in animal products such as meat and dairy, have been linked to an increased risk of diabetes. A meta-analysis of 21 studies including over 347,000 participants found that a higher intake of saturated fats was associated with a 21% increased risk of developing type 2 diabetes compared to a lower intake. The study also found that replacing saturated fats with unsaturated fats, such as those found in nuts, seeds, and vegetable oils, was associated with a lower risk of diabetes.

Trans fats, which are artificially produced by partially hydrogenating vegetable oils to increase their shelf life and stability, are also strongly associated with an increased risk of diabetes. A systematic review and meta-analysis of 17 studies including over 310,000 participants found that a higher intake of trans fats was associated with a 39% increased risk of developing type 2 diabetes compared to a lower intake. The study also found that replacing trans fats with unsaturated fats or whole grains was associated with a lower risk of diabetes.

In contrast, unsaturated fats, which are liquid at room temperature and mainly found in plant-based sources such as nuts, seeds, avocados, and vegetable oils, have been associated with a lower risk of diabetes. A meta-analysis of 20 studies including over 347,000 participants found that a higher intake of unsaturated fats was associated with a 15% lower risk of developing type 2 diabetes compared to a lower intake. The study also found that replacing saturated fats with unsaturated fats was associated with a lower risk of diabetes.

Omega-3 fatty acids, a type of unsaturated fat found in fatty fish, flaxseeds, and walnuts, have also been associated with a lower risk of diabetes. A systematic review and meta-analysis of 10 studies including over 400,000 participants found that a higher intake of omega-3 fatty acids was associated with a 9% lower risk of developing type 2 diabetes compared to a lower intake.

In conclusion, the evidence supports that certain types of fats and oils can increase the risk of developing diabetes, specifically saturated and trans fats. In contrast, unsaturated fats, including omega-3 fatty acids, have been associated with a lower risk of diabetes. Therefore, it is recommended to limit the intake of saturated and trans fats and replace them with healthier unsaturated fats to reduce the risk of developing diabetes. It's important to note that while dietary fats play a role in diabetes risk, other lifestyle factors such as physical activity, maintaining a healthy weight, and avoiding smoking are also critical in diabetes prevention.

18. How does physical activity affect blood sugar levels in people with diabetes?

Physical activity is known to have a significant impact on blood sugar levels, especially in people with diabetes. Regular exercise can help regulate blood sugar levels, improve insulin sensitivity, and reduce the risk of complications associated with diabetes. Here, we will explore how physical activity affects blood sugar levels in people with diabetes, supported by statistical proof and realistic answers.

Physical activity has a direct effect on blood sugar levels by increasing the body's demand for glucose. When we exercise, our muscles require energy to move, which comes from the breakdown of glucose. As a result, the body releases stored glucose from the liver, which raises blood sugar levels. In response to this, the pancreas releases insulin, which allows glucose to enter cells, where it is used for energy. The end result is a decrease in blood sugar levels.

However, the effect of physical activity on blood sugar levels can vary depending on several factors, such as the type and intensity of exercise, the duration of exercise, and the person's overall health status. For example, high-intensity exercise can cause a rapid drop in blood sugar levels, while low-intensity exercise can have a more gradual effect. Moreover, physical activity can also affect blood sugar levels differently in people with different types of diabetes. For instance, people with type 1 diabetes may experience a sudden drop in blood sugar levels during or after exercise, while people with type 2 diabetes may have a slower response.

Several studies have shown that physical activity can improve blood sugar control in people with diabetes. One study published in the Journal of the American Medical Association found that regular exercise was associated with a significant decrease in hemoglobin A1c levels, which is a marker of long-term blood sugar control. The study also found that exercise was associated with a reduction in the need for diabetes medications.

Another study published in Diabetes Care found that a single session of aerobic exercise, such as cycling or walking, improved insulin sensitivity in people with type 2 diabetes. The study also found that exercise reduced the amount of glucose released by the liver, which is a common problem in people with type 2 diabetes.

Realistic answers on how physical activity affects blood sugar levels in people with diabetes

While physical activity can have a positive impact on blood sugar control in people with diabetes, it is essential to approach exercise with caution and consult with a healthcare provider before starting a new exercise program. People with diabetes may need to monitor their blood sugar levels more frequently during and after exercise to ensure they do not experience hypoglycemia (low blood sugar).

Additionally, it is crucial to consider the timing and intensity of exercise to avoid potential complications. For example, people with type 1 diabetes who take insulin may need to adjust their insulin dosage to avoid hypoglycemia during or after exercise. People with diabetic retinopathy or other diabetes-related complications may need to avoid high-impact activities, such as running or jumping, to prevent further damage.

In conclusion, physical activity can have a positive impact on blood sugar control in people with diabetes. However, it is essential to approach exercise with caution and to consult with a healthcare provider before starting a new exercise program. By incorporating regular exercise into their daily routine, people with diabetes can improve their overall health and reduce the risk of complications associated with diabetes.

19. Can certain types of medications increase the risk of developing diabetes, and if so, which ones?

Yes, certain medications can increase the risk of developing diabetes. Some medications can interfere with insulin sensitivity or affect blood glucose levels, leading to an increased risk of developing diabetes or worsening glycemic control in people with pre-existing diabetes. I will discuss some of the medications that have been associated with an increased risk of diabetes.

Glucocorticoids: Glucocorticoids are a type of steroid hormone that is commonly used to treat inflammation, allergies, and autoimmune disorders. They can cause insulin resistance, which can lead to an increased risk of developing type 2 diabetes. The risk of developing diabetes is higher in people taking high doses of glucocorticoids or those taking them for prolonged periods.

Anti-psychotic medications: Anti-psychotic medications are used to treat psychiatric disorders such as schizophrenia and bipolar disorder. They have been associated with an increased risk of developing type 2 diabetes due to their effect on insulin resistance. Anti-psychotic medications that have been linked to an increased risk of diabetes include olanzapine, clozapine, and risperidone.

Beta-blockers: Beta-blockers are commonly used to treat high blood pressure, angina, and heart failure. They have been associated with an increased risk of developing diabetes due to their effect on insulin resistance. Beta-blockers that have been linked to an increased risk of diabetes include propranolol and metoprolol.

Statins: Statins are commonly used to treat high cholesterol levels. They have been associated with an increased risk of developing diabetes, although the risk is small. Statins that have been linked to an increased risk of diabetes include atorvastatin and simvastatin.

Thiazide diuretics: Thiazide diuretics are commonly used to treat high blood pressure. They have been associated with an increased risk of developing diabetes due to their effect on insulin resistance. Thiazide diuretics that have been linked to an increased risk of diabetes include hydrochlorothiazide and chlorthalidone.

Immuno-suppressive medications: Immuno-suppressive medications are commonly used to prevent rejection after an organ transplant or to treat autoimmune disorders. They have been associated with an increased risk of developing diabetes due to their effect on insulin resistance. Immuno-suppressive medications that have been linked to an increased risk of diabetes include cyclosporine and tacrolimus.

It is important to note that not everyone who takes these medications will develop diabetes. The risk of developing diabetes depends on several factors, including age, family history of diabetes, obesity, and lifestyle factors such as diet and exercise. If you are taking any of these medications, it is important to talk to your healthcare provider about your risk of developing diabetes and to discuss strategies to manage your blood glucose levels.

Definitely, certain medications can increase the risk of developing diabetes. Glucocorticoids, anti-psychotic medications, beta-blockers, statins, thiazide diuretics, and immuno-suppressive medications have all been associated with an increased risk of diabetes.

20. What is the link between sleep and diabetes, and how does sleep quality affect blood sugar levels?

There is a strong link between sleep and diabetes. Research has consistently shown that poor sleep quality and quantity can lead to insulin resistance, a key factor in the development of type 2 diabetes. In fact, studies have suggested that people who consistently get less than six hours of sleep per night are at a higher risk of developing diabetes.

Insulin is a hormone produced by the pancreas that regulates blood sugar levels by allowing glucose to enter the body's cells for energy. When the body becomes resistant to insulin, glucose cannot enter the cells effectively, resulting in high blood sugar levels. Over time, this can lead to type 2 diabetes.

Poor sleep quality and quantity can lead to insulin resistance in several ways. One theory is that sleep deprivation can cause the body to release stress hormones, such as cortisol, which can interfere with insulin's ability to regulate blood sugar levels. Additionally, poor sleep can disrupt the body's circadian rhythm, the natural 24-hour cycle that controls various physiological processes, including insulin production and glucose metabolism.

Furthermore, sleep disturbances such as sleep apnea, a condition where breathing stops and starts during sleep, can contribute to the development of diabetes. Sleep apnea has been linked to insulin resistance, and people with diabetes are more likely to have sleep apnea than those without.

Research has also shown that improving sleep quality can lead to better blood sugar control in people with diabetes. A study published in the journal Diabetes Care found that people with type 2 diabetes who participated in a sleep intervention program that included education on sleep hygiene and sleep apnea management saw improvements in their blood sugar levels.

It is essential to maintain good sleep hygiene to improve the quality of sleep. This includes sticking to a regular sleep schedule, avoiding caffeine and alcohol before bedtime, and creating a relaxing sleep environment. For people with sleep apnea, treatments such as continuous positive airway pressure (CPAP) therapy can help improve sleep quality and reduce the risk of developing diabetes.

21. What is the best way to balance protein intake for people with diabetes?

Protein intake is an essential aspect of a healthy diet for people with diabetes. Protein helps regulate blood sugar levels, promotes satiety, and aids in the maintenance of lean body mass. However, it is crucial to balance protein intake to prevent complications associated with diabetes, such as kidney damage.

The American Diabetes Association (ADA) recommends that people with diabetes consume 0.8-1.2 grams of protein per kilogram of body weight per day. For example, a person weighing 68 kg (150 pounds) would need to consume 54-81 grams of protein per day.

Here are some tips on how to balance protein intake for people with diabetes:

Choose lean protein sources: Lean protein sources are low in saturated fat and calories, making them an excellent choice for people with diabetes. Examples of lean protein sources include skinless poultry, fish, lean meat, low-fat dairy, beans, and lentils.

Consider plant-based protein sources: Plant-based protein sources, such as beans, lentils, tofu, and nuts, are excellent options for people with diabetes. These foods are high in fiber and help regulate blood sugar levels.

Watch portion sizes: It is essential to watch portion sizes when consuming protein, as overconsumption can lead to kidney damage. A portion size of protein is typically 3-4 ounces, or the size of a deck of cards.

Limit high-fat protein sources: High-fat protein sources, such as fatty meats, full-fat dairy, and fried foods, should be limited, as they can contribute to weight gain and increase the risk of heart disease.

Spread protein intake throughout the day: Consuming protein throughout the day, rather than in one or two large meals, can help regulate blood sugar levels and promote satiety.

Consult with a registered dietitian: A registered dietitian can help develop a personalized meal plan that balances protein intake with other essential nutrients, such as carbohydrates and fats.

In point of fact, balancing protein intake is crucial for people with diabetes to prevent complications and maintain good health. By choosing lean protein sources, watching portion sizes, and spreading protein intake throughout the day, people with diabetes can enjoy the benefits of protein without putting their health at risk.

22. How does smoking affect the risk of developing diabetes?

Smoking has numerous adverse effects on human health. It is widely known that smoking increases the risk of various health problems, including cardiovascular diseases, respiratory diseases, and cancer. However, smoking also has a negative impact on glucose metabolism and can lead to the development of type 2 diabetes.

Type 2 diabetes is a metabolic disorder characterized by high levels of glucose in the blood. The disease occurs when the body becomes resistant to insulin or does not produce enough insulin to maintain normal blood glucose levels. Smoking affects glucose metabolism in several ways, which can increase the risk of developing type 2 diabetes.

Firstly, smoking causes oxidative stress and inflammation, which can lead to insulin resistance. Oxidative stress occurs when the body is unable to neutralize harmful molecules called free radicals. Free radicals cause damage to cells, including the cells that produce insulin. This damage leads to inflammation, which further impairs insulin sensitivity, making it difficult for the body to regulate glucose levels.

Secondly, smoking can cause endothelial dysfunction, which is a precursor to type 2 diabetes. Endothelial dysfunction is a condition where the lining of the blood vessels is damaged. This damage can reduce the blood flow to the pancreas, which produces insulin, and lead to impaired insulin secretion. Furthermore, smoking can also lead to the accumulation of fat deposits in the pancreas, which can impair its function and contribute to the development of diabetes.

Thirdly, smoking can cause weight gain, which is a significant risk factor for type 2 diabetes. Nicotine in cigarettes increases the release of adrenaline, which suppresses appetite and can lead to temporary weight loss. However, over time, smoking can lead to weight gain, especially in the abdominal region. This type of fat accumulation is associated with insulin resistance and an increased risk of developing type 2 diabetes.

Several studies have shown that smokers are at a higher risk of developing type 2 diabetes compared to non-smokers. For example, a meta-analysis of 25 studies found that current smokers had a 37% increased risk of developing type 2 diabetes compared to non-smokers. Furthermore, the risk of developing diabetes increased with the number of cigarettes smoked per day.

Smoking is a significant risk factor for type 2 diabetes. It can impair glucose metabolism through oxidative stress, inflammation, endothelial dysfunction, and weight gain. Therefore, quitting smoking is one of the most effective ways to reduce the risk of developing diabetes, as well as other health problems associated with smoking.

23. Is diabetes contagious, and if not, how is it transmitted?

Diabetes is not contagious, which means it cannot be transmitted from one person to another like an infectious disease. Instead, diabetes is a metabolic disorder that affects the body's ability to produce or use insulin, a hormone that regulates blood sugar levels.

However, there are some risk factors for type 2 diabetes that may increase the likelihood of developing the condition. These include:

Family history of diabetes

Obesity or being overweight

Sedentary lifestyle

High blood pressure

High cholesterol

Gestational diabetes (diabetes during pregnancy)

Polycystic ovary syndrome (PCOS)

Age (risk increases after age 45)

Race/ethnicity (African Americans, Hispanic/Latinos, Native Americans, and Asian Americans are at higher risk)

24. What are the environmental factors that can increase the risk of developing diabetes?

While genetics plays a significant role in the development of diabetes, environmental factors also contribute to its onset. Let's examine some of them.

Obesity: Being overweight or obese is one of the most significant risk factors for diabetes. Excess body fat can make it more difficult for the body to use insulin effectively, leading to insulin resistance and ultimately, diabetes. According to the Centers for Disease Control and Prevention (CDC), being overweight or obese is the leading risk factor for type 2 diabetes, which accounts for 90-95% of all diabetes cases.

Physical inactivity: Regular physical activity is essential for maintaining a healthy weight and preventing diabetes. Exercise helps the body use insulin more efficiently, which can lower blood sugar levels. Conversely, a sedentary lifestyle can increase the risk of diabetes, even in people who are not overweight. According to the American Diabetes Association, regular physical activity can reduce the risk of diabetes by up to 50%.

Diet: The food we eat plays a crucial role in diabetes prevention. A diet high in processed foods, saturated fats, and added sugars can increase the risk of diabetes. On the other hand, a diet rich in fruits, vegetables, whole grains, and lean protein can help prevent diabetes. According to the CDC, a healthy diet can reduce the risk of diabetes by up to 30%.

Air pollution: Recent research has linked exposure to air pollution with an increased risk of diabetes. Air pollution can trigger inflammation and oxidative stress in the body, both of which can contribute to the development of diabetes. According to a study published in The Lancet Planetary Health, exposure to air pollution was associated with a 21% increase in the risk of diabetes.

Sleep disturbances: Chronic sleep deprivation or poor sleep quality can increase the risk of diabetes. Sleep deprivation can disrupt the body's insulin sensitivity, leading to insulin resistance and ultimately, diabetes. According to a study published in the journal Diabetologia, people who slept less than six hours per night had a 33% higher risk of developing diabetes than those who slept seven to eight hours per night.

25. What are some common misconceptions about diabetes, and how can they be corrected?

Diabetes is a chronic disease that affects millions of people worldwide. Despite its prevalence, there are still many misconceptions surrounding diabetes. These misconceptions can lead to stigma, discrimination, and inadequate care for those living with the disease. Let's explore some common misconceptions about diabetes and provide verified information on how to correct them.

Misconception 1: Diabetes is caused by eating too much sugar.

One of the most common misconceptions about diabetes is that it is caused by eating too much sugar. While consuming too much sugar can lead to weight gain and increase the risk of developing type 2 diabetes, it is not the direct cause of the disease. Diabetes is a complex condition that is caused by a combination of genetic, lifestyle, and environmental factors.

Correcting the misconception: Educate people that while consuming too much sugar may increase the risk of developing type 2 diabetes, it is not the sole cause of the disease.

Misconception 2: Only overweight or obese people develop diabetes.

Another common misconception about diabetes is that only overweight or obese people develop the disease. While being overweight or obese is a risk factor for developing type 2 diabetes, people of all body sizes can develop diabetes.

Correcting the misconception: Educate people that diabetes can affect anyone, regardless of their body size or weight.

Misconception 3: People with diabetes cannot eat any sugar.

Another common misconception is that people with diabetes cannot eat any sugar. While people with diabetes need to manage their blood sugar levels carefully, they can still enjoy sugary foods in moderation as part of a healthy and balanced diet.

Correcting the misconception: Educate people that people with diabetes can still eat sugar in moderation as part of a healthy and balanced diet.

Misconception 4: Diabetes is not a serious disease.

Some people may believe that diabetes is not a serious disease, but this is far from the truth. Diabetes can lead to serious complications, such as heart disease, stroke, kidney failure, and blindness if left unmanaged.

Correcting the misconception: Educate people on the potential complications of diabetes and emphasize the importance of managing the disease to prevent these complications.

Misconception 5: People with diabetes should not exercise.

Finally, some people may believe that people with diabetes should not exercise, but this is not true. Exercise is essential for managing diabetes as it can help to lower blood sugar levels, improve insulin sensitivity, and reduce the risk of complications.

Correcting the misconception: Educate people on the importance of exercise for managing diabetes and encourage people with diabetes to engage in regular physical activity.

In conclusion, there are several common misconceptions about diabetes that can lead to stigma, discrimination, and inadequate care for those living with the disease. By educating people on the facts about diabetes, we can correct these misconceptions and provide better support for those living with the condition.

SECTION 2

TREATMENT OPTIONS

26. What are the treatment options for diabetes?

While there is no cure for diabetes, there are a variety of treatment options available that can help manage the condition and reduce the risk of complications.

The main goals of diabetes treatment are to control blood sugar levels, manage symptoms, and prevent long-term health complications. The treatment options for diabetes vary depending on the type of diabetes, the severity of the condition, and the individual's health and lifestyle factors. Here are some common treatment options for diabetes:

Lifestyle changes: For many people with diabetes, lifestyle changes such as eating a healthy diet, exercising regularly, and losing weight can help manage blood sugar levels and reduce the risk of complications. Quitting smoking and reducing alcohol intake can also be beneficial.

Medications: There are several medications available to treat diabetes, including insulin, which is used to manage Type 1 diabetes, and oral medications such as metformin, sulfonylureas, and meglitinides, which are used to manage Type 2 diabetes.

Blood sugar monitoring: People with diabetes often need to monitor their blood sugar levels regularly using a glucose meter. This can help them keep track of their blood sugar levels and make adjustments to their treatment plan as needed.

Continuous glucose monitoring: This involves wearing a device that continuously monitors blood sugar levels, providing real-time data to help manage diabetes more effectively.

Insulin pumps: These small devices deliver insulin continuously, helping to regulate blood sugar levels more effectively than injections.

Bariatric surgery: In some cases, bariatric surgery may be recommended for people with Type 2 diabetes who are severely overweight. This surgery can help improve blood sugar control and reduce the risk of complications.

It is important to note that diabetes treatment is not a one-size-fits-all approach. Treatment plans should be individualized to meet the unique needs of each person with diabetes. People with diabetes should work closely with their healthcare team to develop a personalized treatment plan that takes into account their medical history, lifestyle factors, and other relevant factors. Regular check-ups and monitoring can also help ensure that treatment is effective and adjusted as needed.

27. Can diabetes be managed solely through diet and exercise?

Yes, diabetes can be managed solely through diet and exercise in some cases, but it depends on the individual's type of diabetes and severity of their condition. Type 1 diabetes, which is an autoimmune disease that destroys the insulin-producing cells in the pancreas, requires insulin therapy and cannot be managed solely through diet and exercise. However, type 2 diabetes, which is a metabolic disorder that affects how the body uses insulin, can often be managed through lifestyle changes.

A healthy diet that is low in carbohydrates and high in fiber, protein, and healthy fats can help regulate blood sugar levels in people with type 2 diabetes. Exercise can also help lower blood sugar levels and improve insulin sensitivity. In fact, the American Diabetes Association recommends at least 150 minutes of moderate-intensity exercise per week for people with diabetes.

Research has shown that lifestyle interventions, including diet and exercise, can be effective in managing type 2 diabetes. One study found that a low-carbohydrate diet was more effective at improving glycemic control than a low-fat diet in people with type 2 diabetes. Another study found that a combination of aerobic and resistance exercise improved glycemic control and reduced medication use in people with type 2 diabetes.

However, it is important to note that lifestyle interventions may not work for everyone with type 2 diabetes, and medication may still be necessary to manage blood sugar levels. Additionally, making lifestyle changes can be challenging, and it is important for individuals to have support from healthcare professionals, family, and friends.

In summary, while type 1 diabetes requires insulin therapy and cannot be managed solely through diet and exercise, lifestyle interventions can be effective in managing type 2 diabetes in some cases. A healthy diet and regular exercise can help regulate blood sugar levels, but medication may still be necessary for some individuals. It is important to work with healthcare professionals to develop an individualized treatment plan that addresses the specific needs of each person with diabetes.

28. How does medication help manage diabetes?

Medications can play a crucial role in managing diabetes by controlling blood glucose levels and preventing complications associated with the condition. The most effective medications for diabetes management depend on the type of diabetes and individual patient factors such as age, medical history, and comorbidities. In general, medications used for diabetes management can be classified into several categories, including insulin, oral hypoglycemic agents, and injectable non-insulin medications.

Insulin is a hormone produced by the pancreas that regulates glucose levels in the blood. People with type 1 diabetes require insulin to survive since their body does not produce insulin. Insulin is also used to manage type 2 diabetes when diet, exercise, and oral medications are insufficient in controlling blood glucose levels. Several types of insulin are available, including rapid-acting, short-acting, intermediate-acting, and long-acting. Insulin can be administered using an injection, insulin pen, or insulin pump.

Oral hypoglycemic agents are medications that are taken by mouth to help control blood glucose levels in people with type 2 diabetes. The most commonly prescribed oral medications include metformin, sulfonylureas, meglitinides, and thiazolidinediones. Metformin is the first-line oral medication for most people with type 2 diabetes, as it helps to lower blood glucose levels by reducing glucose production in the liver and increasing glucose uptake by the muscles.

Injectable non-insulin medications are used to manage type 2 diabetes when other medications are not effective or not tolerated. These medications work by increasing insulin production, decreasing glucose production in the liver, and slowing down glucose absorption in the gut. Examples of these medications include GLP-1 receptor agonists and amylin analogs.

Several studies have shown the efficacy of various diabetes medications in managing blood glucose levels and preventing diabetes-related complications. For example, a randomized controlled trial found that metformin reduced the risk of diabetes-related complications such as cardiovascular disease, kidney disease, and nerve damage in people with type 2 diabetes. GLP-1 receptor agonists have also been shown to reduce blood glucose levels and promote weight loss in people with type 2 diabetes.

So, medication can be an essential tool in managing diabetes, and a variety of medications are available depending on the type of diabetes and individual patient factors. Insulin, oral hypoglycemic agents, and injectable non-insulin medications have been shown to effectively control blood glucose levels and reduce the risk of diabetes-related complications. It is essential to work closely with a healthcare professional to determine the best medication regimen for an individual's specific needs and to ensure proper management of their diabetes.

29. What is the role of insulin in diabetes treatment?

Insulin is a hormone produced by the pancreas that helps regulate blood sugar levels in the body. In diabetes, the body is either unable to produce enough insulin or is unable to use insulin effectively, resulting in high blood sugar levels. Insulin therapy is a cornerstone of diabetes treatment and is used to replace the deficient insulin or increase insulin levels in the body.

The primary goal of insulin therapy in diabetes treatment is to regulate blood sugar levels and prevent complications associated with high blood sugar levels, such as damage to blood vessels, nerves, and organs. Insulin therapy is typically prescribed for individuals with type 1 diabetes, a condition in which the pancreas does not produce insulin, or type 2 diabetes, a condition in which the body becomes resistant to insulin.

Insulin therapy can be delivered through injections or an insulin pump, which delivers insulin continuously through a small tube placed under the skin. The type and dose of insulin used depend on various factors, including the individual's blood sugar levels, lifestyle, and other medical conditions.

Insulin therapy has several benefits, including improved blood sugar control, reduced risk of complications, and improved quality of life. However, it can also have side effects, such as low blood sugar levels, weight gain, and injection site reactions.

Insulin therapy is typically used in conjunction with other diabetes treatments, including lifestyle modifications such as a healthy diet, regular exercise, and weight management. In some cases, oral medications may also be prescribed to help regulate blood sugar levels.

Therefore, insulin therapy plays a crucial role in diabetes treatment by regulating blood sugar levels and preventing complications associated with high blood sugar levels. Insulin therapy is a safe and effective treatment option for individuals with diabetes and should be used in conjunction with other diabetes treatments, including lifestyle modifications and oral medications, to achieve optimal blood sugar control and improve overall health outcomes.

30. Can diabetes be cured?

Diabetes is a chronic condition that affects the way the body processes glucose (sugar), resulting in high blood sugar levels. There are two main types of diabetes: type 1 and type 2.

Type 1 diabetes is an autoimmune disorder where the body's immune system attacks the cells in the pancreas that produce insulin. Insulin is necessary for the body to process glucose, so people with type 1 diabetes require insulin injections to regulate their blood sugar levels. Type 1 diabetes cannot be cured, but it can be managed through insulin therapy and lifestyle changes.

Type 2 diabetes, on the other hand, is a metabolic disorder that occurs when the body becomes resistant to insulin or doesn't produce enough insulin. Type 2 diabetes is often linked to obesity and lifestyle factors such as diet and exercise. While type 2 diabetes cannot be cured, it can be managed through lifestyle changes, medication, and insulin therapy in some cases.

While there is currently no cure for diabetes, there is ongoing research into potential treatments and ways to prevent the development of diabetes. For example, a study published in the Lancet Diabetes and Endocrinology found that weight loss and lifestyle changes, such as following a healthy diet and increasing physical activity, can help put type 2 diabetes into remission for some individuals.

It's important to note that managing diabetes is a lifelong commitment, and people with diabetes need to monitor their blood sugar levels regularly and make adjustments to their diet, medication, and lifestyle as needed. While there is no cure, with proper management, people with diabetes can lead healthy, active lives.

31. What are the potential side effects of diabetes medication?

The goal of diabetes medication is to help manage blood sugar levels and prevent complications from the disease. While diabetes medication can be effective in achieving these goals, they can also have potential side effects. We will discuss some common side effects associated with different types of diabetes medications.

Metformin: Metformin is a commonly used medication for type 2 diabetes. It works by reducing the amount of glucose produced by the liver and increasing the body's sensitivity to insulin. Some potential side effects of metformin include gastrointestinal issues such as nausea, diarrhea, and abdominal pain. In rare cases, metformin can also cause lactic acidosis, a serious condition that can lead to organ damage.

Sulfonylureas: Sulfonylureas are a class of medications that help the pancreas produce more insulin. Common sulfonylureas include glipizide, glyburide, and glimepiride. One potential side effect of sulfonylureas is hypoglycemia (low blood sugar). Symptoms of hypoglycemia can include dizziness, confusion, and fatigue. Sulfonylureas can also cause weight gain and an increased risk of cardiovascular events.

DPP-4 inhibitors: DPP-4 inhibitors are a newer class of diabetes medication that help regulate blood sugar levels by blocking the action of an enzyme that breaks down incretin hormones. These hormones increase insulin secretion and decrease glucose production. Some potential side effects of DPP-4 inhibitors include upper respiratory tract infections, headaches, and joint pain.

SGLT2 inhibitors: SGLT2 inhibitors are a class of medication that help lower blood sugar levels by preventing the kidneys from reabsorbing glucose. Potential side effects of SGLT2 inhibitors include genital yeast infections, urinary tract infections, and an increased risk of diabetic ketoacidosis (DKA), a serious condition that can lead to coma or death.

It's important to note that not all diabetes medications cause side effects, and not all people will experience the same side effects. Additionally, some people may be more likely to experience certain side effects based on their age, gender, and other health conditions. If you're experiencing side effects from your diabetes medication, talk to your healthcare provider about adjusting your treatment plan. They may be able to recommend a different medication or dosage that better meets your needs.

32. How often should blood sugar levels be monitored?

The frequency of monitoring blood sugar levels depends on several factors, including the individual's health status, the type of diabetes they have, their treatment plan, and their lifestyle.

For individuals with type 1 diabetes, blood sugar levels should be monitored frequently, at least four times a day. This is because individuals with type 1 diabetes do not produce insulin, and therefore they need to closely monitor their blood sugar levels to ensure they are within a healthy range. Frequent monitoring is necessary to avoid the complications associated with high or low blood sugar levels, such as diabetic ketoacidosis (DKA) or hypoglycemia.

For individuals with type 2 diabetes, the frequency of monitoring blood sugar levels can vary depending on their treatment plan and how well their blood sugar levels are controlled. If an individual is managing their diabetes with lifestyle changes, such as diet and exercise, they may only need to monitor their blood sugar levels a few times a week. However, if an individual is taking medication or insulin to manage their diabetes, they may need to monitor their blood sugar levels more frequently, at least once or twice a day.

Pregnant women with gestational diabetes need to monitor their blood sugar levels regularly to ensure that their blood sugar levels are within a healthy range for both the mother and the baby. They may need to check their blood sugar levels before and after meals, and possibly at bedtime.

Individuals with prediabetes may not need to monitor their blood sugar levels as frequently as those with diabetes. However, regular monitoring can help them identify changes in their blood sugar levels and make lifestyle changes to prevent the development of diabetes.

Summarily, the frequency of monitoring blood sugar levels varies depending on the individual's health status, the type of diabetes they have, their treatment plan, and their lifestyle. It is important to follow the advice of a healthcare professional regarding how often to monitor blood sugar levels to ensure optimal diabetes management and reduce the risk of complications associated with high or low blood sugar levels.

33. What is the best way to manage blood sugar levels?

Maintaining healthy blood sugar levels is essential for overall health and well-being, as high blood sugar levels can lead to various health complications like diabetes, heart disease, and nerve damage. Here are some effective ways to manage blood sugar levels:

Follow a healthy diet: A healthy diet can help control blood sugar levels by regulating the amount and timing of carbohydrate intake. A balanced diet should include whole grains, fruits, vegetables, lean proteins, and healthy fats.

Exercise regularly: Regular physical activity can help lower blood sugar levels by increasing insulin sensitivity. Aim for at least 30 minutes of moderate-intensity exercise five days a week.

Monitor blood sugar levels: Regular monitoring of blood sugar levels can help identify any fluctuations and allow for prompt management. Blood sugar levels should be monitored as recommended by a healthcare professional.

Take medications as prescribed: If prescribed medication for diabetes, it is important to take them as directed by your healthcare provider. Skipping doses or not taking medication as prescribed can lead to uncontrolled blood sugar levels.

Get enough sleep: Adequate sleep is essential for good health, and studies have shown that insufficient sleep can lead to insulin resistance and higher blood sugar levels.

Manage stress: Chronic stress can increase blood sugar levels by triggering the release of stress hormones. Find healthy ways to manage stress, such as meditation, deep breathing exercises, or talking to a therapist.

Maintain a healthy weight: Obesity is a risk factor for diabetes, and losing weight can help improve insulin sensitivity and regulate blood sugar levels.

34. Is weight loss beneficial for diabetes management?

Weight loss can be a beneficial tool for managing diabetes, particularly type 2 diabetes, as it can improve blood glucose control and reduce the risk of diabetes-related complications. Here are some verified pieces of information and realistic answers regarding weight loss and diabetes management:

Weight loss can help improve insulin sensitivity: Insulin is a hormone that regulates blood glucose levels in the body. In people with type 2 diabetes, the body becomes resistant to insulin, and the pancreas is unable to produce enough insulin to compensate for this resistance. Losing weight can help improve insulin sensitivity, which means the body is better able to use the insulin it produces.

Weight loss can lower blood glucose levels: When the body is carrying excess weight, it can be harder for insulin to do its job, which can result in higher blood glucose levels. Losing weight can help lower blood glucose levels, making it easier to manage diabetes.

Weight loss can reduce the risk of diabetes-related complications: People with diabetes are at a higher risk of developing complications such as heart disease, stroke, kidney disease, and nerve damage. Losing weight can help reduce the risk of these complications and improve overall health.

Weight loss should be approached in a healthy and sustainable way: Crash diets or extreme calorie restriction can be harmful to overall health and may not result in long-term weight loss. A healthy weight loss approach involves making gradual changes to diet and exercise habits and setting realistic goals.

Consultation with a healthcare provider is essential: It is important to consult with a healthcare provider before starting any weight loss program, particularly if you have diabetes. Your healthcare provider can help you determine a safe and realistic weight loss goal and provide guidance on the best approach for you.

In general, weight loss can be beneficial for diabetes management, but it should be approached in a healthy and sustainable way with the guidance of a healthcare provider. Losing weight can improve insulin sensitivity, lower blood glucose levels, and reduce the risk of diabetes-related complications. However, it is important to set realistic goals and make gradual changes to diet and exercise habits to achieve long-term success.

35. Are there any natural remedies that can help manage diabetes?

Diabetes is a chronic metabolic disorder characterized by high blood glucose levels due to insufficient insulin production or insulin resistance. While there is no cure for diabetes, there are natural remedies that can help manage the condition. Here are some natural remedies for managing diabetes that have been supported by scientific research:

Diet modification: Eating a balanced diet can help manage blood glucose levels. A diet rich in fiber, whole grains, fruits, and vegetables can help control blood sugar levels, improve insulin sensitivity, and reduce the risk of diabetes-related complications.

Exercise: Regular exercise can help lower blood glucose levels by increasing insulin sensitivity. Exercise also promotes weight loss, which can help control blood sugar levels in people with type 2 diabetes.

Cinnamon: Cinnamon has been shown to improve insulin sensitivity, which can help manage blood sugar levels. Studies have suggested that consuming 1-6 grams of cinnamon per day can significantly reduce fasting blood glucose levels.

Chromium: Chromium is a mineral that plays a role in insulin action and glucose metabolism. Studies have suggested that taking chromium supplements can improve glucose tolerance and reduce insulin resistance.

Omega-3 fatty acids: Omega-3 fatty acids, found in fatty fish, nuts, and seeds, can help reduce inflammation and improve insulin sensitivity. Studies have suggested that consuming omega-3 fatty acids can help lower fasting blood glucose levels and reduce the risk of diabetes-related complications.

It is important to note that while these natural remedies can help manage diabetes, they should not be used as a substitute for medical treatment. People with diabetes should always consult with their healthcare provider before trying any natural remedies or making significant changes to their diet or exercise routine. Additionally, natural remedies may not work for everyone, and people with diabetes should continue to monitor their blood glucose levels and follow their healthcare provider's recommendations for managing their condition.

36. Can protein and fat intake affect blood sugar levels in diabetes?

Yes, both protein and fat intake can affect blood sugar levels in diabetes, but the effect may vary depending on the type and amount of each nutrient consumed.

Protein intake can affect blood sugar levels in people with diabetes, but the effect is usually less significant than that of carbohydrates. Protein is broken down into amino acids, which can be converted into glucose in the liver through a process called gluconeogenesis. However, the rate of gluconeogenesis is generally slower and more stable than the breakdown of carbohydrates, leading to a more gradual rise in blood sugar levels. Furthermore, protein also stimulates the release of insulin, which can help lower blood sugar levels. Therefore, a moderate amount of protein intake (about 15-20% of total daily calories) is generally recommended for people with diabetes to help maintain blood sugar levels.

Fat intake can also affect blood sugar levels in people with diabetes, but the effect is more complex and less well-understood than that of carbohydrates or protein. Some types of fat, such as monounsaturated and polyunsaturated fats, can have a beneficial effect on blood sugar levels by improving insulin sensitivity and reducing inflammation. On the other hand, saturated and trans fats can have a negative effect on blood sugar levels by impairing insulin sensitivity and increasing inflammation. Additionally, high-fat meals can delay stomach emptying and slow down the absorption of carbohydrates, leading to a more gradual rise in blood sugar levels. Therefore, it is recommended that people with diabetes consume a moderate amount of healthy fats (such as avocados, nuts, and fatty fish) and limit their intake of saturated and trans fats (such as red meat and processed foods).

37. What foods should be avoided for people with diabetes?

People with diabetes need to manage their diet carefully to maintain healthy blood sugar levels. While there are no specific foods that people with diabetes must avoid entirely, there are some foods that they should limit or avoid to prevent spikes in blood sugar levels. Here are some examples:

Sugary foods and drinks: Foods and drinks high in added sugars should be avoided or limited as they can cause blood sugar levels to rise quickly. This includes soda, juice, candy, cakes, cookies, and other sweets.

Carbohydrates: Carbohydrates are broken down into glucose during digestion and can cause blood sugar levels to spike. People with diabetes should limit their intake of refined carbohydrates such as white bread, pasta, and rice. Instead, they should opt for complex carbohydrates found in whole grains, fruits, and vegetables.

Saturated and Trans Fats: Foods high in saturated and trans fats, such as fried foods, processed meats, and high-fat dairy products, can contribute to the development of insulin resistance, which can make it harder for the body to control blood sugar levels.

Alcohol: Alcohol can cause blood sugar levels to fluctuate, and it can also interfere with diabetes medications. People with diabetes should limit their alcohol intake and always drink in moderation.

Processed Foods: Processed foods are often high in salt, sugar, and unhealthy fats, all of which can contribute to the development of diabetes and make it harder to manage blood sugar levels. People with diabetes should opt for fresh, whole foods instead.

It's important to note that there is no one-size-fits-all approach to diabetes management. Each person with diabetes should work with their healthcare team to develop a personalized eating plan that meets their specific needs and goals. Additionally, maintaining a healthy weight, staying physically active, and taking any prescribed medications are also important components of diabetes management.

38. What are some healthy food options for people with diabetes?

Diabetes is a chronic medical condition that requires careful management of one's diet and lifestyle. A healthy and balanced diet is an essential component of diabetes management. It helps regulate blood sugar levels, improve insulin sensitivity, reduce the risk of complications, and promote overall health and wellbeing. Here are some healthy food options for people with diabetes:

Non-Starchy Vegetables: Vegetables are low in calories and high in fiber, vitamins, and minerals. Non-starchy vegetables such as leafy greens, broccoli, cauliflower, carrots, and bell peppers are excellent choices for people with diabetes. They have a low glycemic index and can help regulate blood sugar levels.

Whole Grains: Whole grains such as brown rice, quinoa, whole wheat, and oats are excellent sources of fiber, which can help regulate blood sugar levels and improve insulin sensitivity. They are also rich in vitamins and minerals, making them a healthy option for people with diabetes.

Lean Proteins: Lean proteins such as skinless chicken, turkey, fish, tofu, and legumes are excellent sources of protein and do not contain added sugars or saturated fats. They can help regulate blood sugar levels and promote satiety, which can help prevent overeating.

Low-Fat Dairy: Low-fat dairy products such as skim milk, low-fat yogurt, and low-fat cheese are excellent sources of calcium and vitamin D. They are also low in calories and can help regulate blood sugar levels.

Fruits: Fruits are rich in fiber, vitamins, and minerals. However, they also contain natural sugars, which can raise blood sugar levels. It is best to choose fruits with a low glycemic index, such as berries, apples, and oranges, and to eat them in moderation.

Nuts and Seeds: Nuts and seeds such as almonds, walnuts, chia seeds, and flaxseeds are rich in healthy fats, fiber, and protein. They can help regulate blood sugar levels and promote satiety, which can help prevent overeating.

It is important to note that portion control is critical for people with diabetes. It is also essential to limit or avoid foods that are high in added sugars, saturated fats, and refined carbohydrates. Examples include sugary beverages, processed snacks, and fried foods.

39. How can meal planning help manage diabetes?

Meal planning is an essential component of managing diabetes. It helps people with diabetes to make healthier food choices, control blood sugar levels, and maintain a healthy weight. A balanced diet with the right mix of carbohydrates, proteins, and fats can help regulate blood sugar levels and prevent spikes and crashes.

Here are some ways meal planning can help manage diabetes:

Maintain a healthy weight: Being overweight or obese increases the risk of developing type 2 diabetes. Meal planning can help manage diabetes by reducing the risk of weight gain and promoting weight loss. This involves creating a calorie deficit by choosing foods with fewer calories and increasing physical activity.

Control blood sugar levels: Consistency in eating patterns is crucial in regulating blood sugar levels. Meal planning involves spacing meals evenly throughout the day, and choosing foods with a low glycemic index. The glycemic index is a measure of how quickly foods raise blood sugar levels. Foods with a high glycemic index should be limited because they cause blood sugar levels to spike.

Choose healthy foods: Meal planning encourages the consumption of nutrient-rich foods such as fruits, vegetables, whole grains, lean proteins, and healthy fats. These foods provide the necessary nutrients without spiking blood sugar levels. Processed and sugary foods should be avoided or consumed in moderation.

Reduce the risk of complications: Uncontrolled diabetes can lead to several health complications such as heart disease, kidney disease, and nerve damage. Meal planning helps manage diabetes by reducing the risk of these complications. Eating a balanced diet can help regulate blood sugar levels, lower cholesterol, and maintain blood pressure within healthy limits.

Simplify meal preparation: Meal planning involves creating a weekly or monthly meal plan, making a grocery list, and preparing meals in advance. This can simplify meal preparation and reduce the need for takeout or fast food, which may contain high amounts of sugar, salt, and unhealthy fats.

It's important to note that meal planning for diabetes is not a one-size-fits-all approach. The ideal meal plan depends on individual preferences, lifestyle, and health goals. Consultation with a registered dietitian or a certified diabetes educator can help develop a personalized meal plan that works best.

40. What role does exercise play in diabetes management?

Exercise plays a crucial role in diabetes management as it can help to control blood sugar levels, reduce insulin resistance, and lower the risk of developing other health conditions associated with diabetes. Exercise also has numerous additional health benefits, such as improving heart health, reducing stress and anxiety, and promoting weight loss. I will provide verified information and realistic answers regarding the role of exercise in diabetes management.

Exercise and Blood Sugar Control

When you exercise, your muscles use glucose for energy, which can help to lower blood sugar levels. Exercise also helps to improve insulin sensitivity, allowing insulin to be more effective in transporting glucose into cells. This can be especially helpful for people with type 2 diabetes who may have insulin resistance, meaning that their cells do not respond as well to insulin. It is important to note that the effects of exercise on blood sugar can vary depending on the type and intensity of exercise, as well as individual factors such as diet and medication use.

Exercise and Cardiovascular Health

People with diabetes are at a higher risk of developing cardiovascular disease, so exercise can be an important tool for managing this risk. Regular exercise can help to improve heart health by reducing blood pressure and cholesterol levels, as well as reducing the risk of heart attack and stroke.

Exercise and Weight Management

Maintaining a healthy weight is important for managing diabetes, and exercise can be a helpful tool for weight loss and weight management. Regular exercise can help to burn calories and build muscle, which can increase metabolism and help to reduce body fat. Exercise can also help to reduce appetite and cravings, making it easier to stick to a healthy diet.

Realistic Exercise Recommendations for Diabetes Management

The American Diabetes Association recommends that adults with diabetes aim for at least 150 minutes of moderate-intensity aerobic exercise per week, spread out over at least three days. Examples of moderate-intensity exercise include brisk walking, cycling, swimming, or dancing. Strength training exercises, such as lifting weights or using resistance bands, should also be included at least twice a week to build muscle and improve overall fitness.

It is important to start slowly and gradually increase the intensity and duration of exercise, especially for those who are new to exercise or have not exercised in a while. It is also important to monitor blood sugar levels before, during, and after exercise, and to talk to a healthcare professional before starting an exercise program.

41. Can stress management techniques help control blood sugar levels in diabetes?

Stress is a normal part of life, and everyone experiences it from time to time. However, chronic stress can have negative effects on health, including blood sugar levels in people with diabetes. Stress hormones such as cortisol and adrenaline can cause blood sugar levels to rise, leading to potential complications in people with diabetes. Fortunately, stress management techniques can help control blood sugar levels in diabetes. These techniques involve a variety of strategies that help reduce stress and promote relaxation. Here are some of the most effective stress management techniques for diabetes:

Exercise: Regular physical activity can help reduce stress and lower blood sugar levels. Exercise can also help improve insulin sensitivity, making it easier for the body to use insulin and control blood sugar levels.

Meditation: Meditation is a practice that involves focusing your attention on a specific object, thought, or activity to promote relaxation and reduce stress. There is evidence that regular meditation can help lower blood sugar levels in people with diabetes.

Yoga: Yoga is a mind-body practice that combines physical postures, breathing techniques, and meditation. It has been shown to reduce stress and improve blood sugar control in people with diabetes.

Deep breathing: Deep breathing exercises can help reduce stress and lower blood sugar levels. They involve taking slow, deep breaths and exhaling slowly.

Cognitive-behavioral therapy: Cognitive-behavioral therapy is a type of talk therapy that focuses on changing negative thought patterns and behaviors. It has been shown to be effective in reducing stress and improving blood sugar control in people with diabetes.

It is important to note that stress management techniques should be used in conjunction with other diabetes management strategies, such as medication, diet, and regular monitoring of blood sugar levels. It is also important to consult with a healthcare provider before starting any new stress management techniques, especially if you have any medical conditions or are taking medication.

No doubt stress management techniques can help control blood sugar levels in diabetes. These techniques promote relaxation and reduce stress, which can lead to better blood sugar control. Regular exercise, meditation, yoga, deep breathing, and cognitive-behavioral therapy are all effective stress management techniques for diabetes. However, it is important to use these techniques in conjunction with other diabetes management strategies and to consult with a healthcare provider before starting any new stress management techniques.

42. What is the impact of alcohol consumption on diabetes?

Alcohol consumption can have both positive and negative effects on diabetes, depending on the amount and frequency of consumption. The following provides an overview of the impact of alcohol consumption on diabetes, based on verified information from scientific studies.

Positive Effects:

Moderate alcohol consumption has been associated with a reduced risk of type 2 diabetes. According to a study published in the Journal of the American Medical Association (JAMA), moderate alcohol consumption (up to 1 drink per day for women and up to 2 drinks per day for men) was associated with a 30% lower risk of developing type 2 diabetes compared to non-drinkers.

The reason for this may be due to the fact that moderate alcohol consumption has been shown to increase insulin sensitivity and improve glucose metabolism.

Negative Effects:

Heavy alcohol consumption, on the other hand, can have negative effects on diabetes. Heavy drinking can lead to high blood sugar levels, which can make it difficult to manage diabetes. Alcohol is also high in calories and can contribute to weight gain, which is a risk factor for type 2 diabetes.

Furthermore, heavy alcohol consumption can lead to alcoholic liver disease, which can cause insulin resistance and increase the risk of developing type 2 diabetes. A study published in the Journal of Hepatology found that heavy alcohol consumption was associated with an increased risk of developing type 2 diabetes, and that this risk was higher in individuals with alcoholic liver disease. In addition to the negative effects on diabetes, heavy alcohol consumption can also lead to other health problems, including liver disease, heart disease, and cancer.

Therefore, it is important for individuals with diabetes to limit their alcohol consumption and to discuss any concerns with their healthcare provider. It is recommended that men should not have more than 2 drinks per day, and women should not have more than 1 drink per day. Furthermore, it is important to maintain a healthy lifestyle, including a balanced diet, regular exercise, and maintaining a healthy weight to manage diabetes effectively.

43. Can smoking affect diabetes management?

Smoking can significantly affect diabetes management in several ways. Here are some of the ways smoking can impact diabetes:

Increased Risk of Developing Type 2 Diabetes: Smoking can increase the risk of developing type 2 diabetes by up to 40%, according to the Centers for Disease Control and Prevention (CDC). Smoking can lead to insulin resistance, which can make it harder for the body to use insulin effectively and regulate blood sugar levels.

Impaired Blood Sugar Control: Smoking can worsen blood sugar control in people with diabetes. The nicotine in cigarettes can cause blood sugar levels to rise, and smoking can make it harder for insulin to work properly, leading to higher blood sugar levels.

Increased Risk of Diabetes Complications: Smoking can increase the risk of diabetes complications such as heart disease, nerve damage, kidney damage, and vision problems. People with diabetes who smoke are at a higher risk for these complications compared to people with diabetes who do not smoke.

Reduced Effectiveness of Diabetes Medications: Smoking can reduce the effectiveness of some diabetes medications. For example, smoking can decrease the effectiveness of metformin, which is a commonly prescribed medication for type 2 diabetes.

Increased Risk of Hypoglycemia: Smoking can increase the risk of hypoglycemia (low blood sugar) in people with diabetes. This is because smoking can reduce appetite, leading to less food intake, which can cause blood sugar levels to drop.

In addition to these health effects, smoking can also make it harder to manage diabetes in other ways. For example, smoking can make it more difficult to exercise, which is an important part of diabetes management. Smoking can also lead to stress and anxiety, which can make it harder to manage blood sugar levels.

Quitting smoking can have significant benefits for people with diabetes. According to the American Diabetes Association, quitting smoking can improve blood sugar control and reduce the risk of diabetes complications. It can also improve overall health and reduce the risk of other health problems, such as heart disease and cancer.

44. Can diabetes be prevented?

While there is no guaranteed way to prevent diabetes, there are several steps people can take to reduce their risk of developing the condition. One of the most important ways to prevent diabetes is by maintaining a healthy lifestyle. This includes eating a healthy diet that is rich in fruits, vegetables, whole grains, and lean proteins while limiting sugary and processed foods. Regular exercise is also essential to maintaining a healthy weight and reducing the risk of developing diabetes.

Another important factor in preventing diabetes is maintaining a healthy weight. Being overweight or obese is a significant risk factor for developing diabetes. Studies have shown that losing even a small amount of weight, as little as 5-7% of total body weight, can significantly reduce the risk of developing Type 2 diabetes.

In addition to lifestyle factors, there are also some medical treatments that can help prevent diabetes. For example, studies have shown that certain medications, such as metformin, can help reduce the risk of developing Type 2 diabetes in people with prediabetes.

It is also essential to monitor blood sugar levels and get regular check-ups from a healthcare professional, especially if there is a family history of diabetes. Early detection and treatment of diabetes can help prevent complications such as heart disease, nerve damage, and kidney damage.

While there is no guaranteed way to prevent diabetes, adopting a healthy lifestyle and managing risk factors can significantly reduce the risk of developing the condition.

It is essential to consult with a healthcare professional to determine the best course of action for preventing diabetes based on individual risk factors and medical history.

45. What lifestyle changes can help prevent diabetes?

While there are several factors that contribute to the development of diabetes, lifestyle choices play a significant role in the prevention of the disease. Here are some lifestyle changes that can help prevent diabetes:

Maintain a healthy weight: Being overweight or obese is a significant risk factor for diabetes. Studies have shown that losing just 5-10% of your body weight can significantly reduce your risk of developing diabetes. Maintaining a healthy weight through a balanced diet and regular exercise can help prevent diabetes.

Exercise regularly: Regular exercise can help improve insulin sensitivity, which can lower blood sugar levels and reduce the risk of developing diabetes. Aim for at least 30 minutes of moderate-intensity exercise, such as brisk walking or cycling, most days of the week.

Eat a healthy diet: A healthy diet can help prevent diabetes by promoting weight loss, reducing inflammation, and improving insulin sensitivity. Focus on eating a variety of nutrient-dense foods, such as fruits, vegetables, whole grains, lean proteins, and healthy fats. Limit processed foods, sugary drinks, and foods high in saturated and trans fats.

Avoid smoking: Smoking is a significant risk factor for diabetes. Studies have shown that smokers are more likely to develop diabetes than non-smokers. Quitting smoking can significantly reduce your risk of developing diabetes.

Limit alcohol consumption: Excessive alcohol consumption can increase the risk of developing diabetes. Men should limit their alcohol intake to no more than two drinks per day, while women should limit their intake to no more than one drink per day.

Manage stress: Chronic stress can increase the risk of developing diabetes by increasing cortisol levels, which can raise blood sugar levels. Practicing stress-reducing activities such as yoga, meditation, or deep breathing exercises can help manage stress levels.

Get enough sleep: Lack of sleep can disrupt the body's insulin sensitivity, which can increase the risk of developing diabetes. Aim for at least 7-8 hours of sleep per night to promote healthy blood sugar levels.

Making healthy lifestyle choices can significantly reduce the risk of developing diabetes. By maintaining a healthy weight, exercising regularly, eating a healthy diet, avoiding smoking, limiting alcohol consumption, managing stress, and getting enough sleep, you can help prevent diabetes and improve your overall health. Consult with a healthcare professional to create a personalized plan that works for you.

46. Is diabetes a death sentence?

When you have diabetes, your body either doesn't make enough insulin or can't use the insulin it makes as well as it should. This can lead to a buildup of sugar in your bloodstream, which can cause serious health problems if left untreated.

However, having diabetes is not necessarily a death sentence. With proper management, people with diabetes can live long, healthy lives.

Diabetes can be managed through a combination of lifestyle changes, medication, and monitoring blood sugar levels. Here are some things you can do to manage your diabetes:

Maintain a healthy weight: If you're overweight, losing even a small amount of weight can help improve your blood sugar levels.

Eat a healthy diet: Eating a balanced diet that's rich in fruits, vegetables, whole grains, lean protein, and healthy fats can help keep your blood sugar levels stable.

Exercise regularly: Physical activity can help lower blood sugar levels and improve insulin sensitivity.

Take medication as prescribed: If your doctor has prescribed medication to help manage your diabetes, it's important to take it as directed.

Monitor your blood sugar levels: Regular monitoring of your blood sugar levels can help you make adjustments to your diet, exercise, and medication as needed.

While diabetes can lead to serious health problems if left untreated, such as heart disease, stroke, kidney disease, and nerve damage, with proper management, the risk of these complications can be greatly reduced.

It's important to work closely with your healthcare team to develop a diabetes management plan that works for you. This may include regular checkups, blood tests, and medication adjustments as needed.

47. Can people with diabetes live a healthy and normal life expectancy?

Yes, people with diabetes can live a healthy and normal life expectancy with proper management of their condition.

The key to managing diabetes is to keep blood sugar levels within a healthy range. This can be achieved through a combination of medication, diet, exercise, and regular monitoring. People with type 1 diabetes need to take insulin to regulate their blood sugar levels, while people with type 2 diabetes may be able to manage their condition with lifestyle changes and oral medications.

It is important for people with diabetes to make healthy lifestyle choices to help manage their condition. This includes maintaining a healthy weight, eating a balanced diet, and engaging in regular physical activity. Exercise can help to lower blood sugar levels, improve cardiovascular health, and reduce the risk of other health problems such as high blood pressure and high cholesterol.

There are also several potential complications associated with diabetes that can be prevented or managed with proper care. These complications include neuropathy (nerve damage), retinopathy (eye damage), nephropathy (kidney damage), and cardiovascular disease. Regular check-ups with a healthcare provider and monitoring of blood sugar levels can help to prevent or detect these complications early, which can improve outcomes.

The American Diabetes Association recommends that people with diabetes have an A1C test at least twice a year to monitor their blood sugar levels. They should also have their blood pressure, cholesterol, and kidney function checked regularly. Additionally, people with diabetes should receive an annual dilated eye exam to check for any signs of retinopathy.

In conclusion, people with diabetes can live a healthy and normal life expectancy with proper management of their condition. This includes making healthy lifestyle choices, monitoring blood sugar levels, and receiving regular check-ups with a healthcare provider. With proper care, people with diabetes can reduce the risk of complications and enjoy a full and active life.

48. Can the intake of bitter substance mitigate against diabetes?

Bitter substances, such as bitter melon, bitter gourd, and neem, have been traditionally used as medicinal plants to treat various ailments, including diabetes. The bitter taste is due to the presence of compounds known as bitter principles, which have been shown to have anti-diabetic properties.

Bitter melon, also known as bitter gourd or Momordica charantia, is a fruit that is commonly used as a food and traditional medicine in Asia, Africa, and South America. It contains several bioactive compounds, including charantin, vicine, and polypeptide-p, which have been shown to have anti-diabetic properties. Charantin and vicine are believed to lower blood glucose levels by stimulating the release of insulin, while polypeptide-p has insulin-like properties that can lower blood sugar levels.

Several studies have investigated the effectiveness of bitter melon in managing diabetes. A systematic review and meta-analysis of randomized controlled trials found that bitter melon significantly reduced fasting blood glucose levels in patients with type 2 diabetes. Another study found that bitter melon extract improved insulin sensitivity and reduced HbA1c levels in patients with type 2 diabetes.

Neem, also known as Azadirachta indica, is a tree that is native to India and Southeast Asia. Its leaves, seeds, and bark have been used in traditional medicine to treat various ailments, including diabetes. Neem contains several bioactive compounds, including flavonoids, triterpenoids, and glycosides, which have been shown to have anti-diabetic properties.

Several studies have investigated the effectiveness of neem in managing diabetes. A randomized controlled trial found that neem leaf extract significantly reduced fasting blood glucose levels in patients with type 2 diabetes. Another study found that neem leaf extract improved insulin sensitivity and reduced HbA1c levels in patients with type 2 diabetes.

Despite the promising results of these studies, more research is needed to determine the optimal dose, duration, and safety of bitter substances for managing diabetes. Bitter substances can have side effects, such as gastrointestinal upset, and may interact with medications, so it is important to consult with a healthcare provider before using them as a treatment for diabetes.

In conclusion, bitter substances such as bitter melon and neem have shown promising results in managing diabetes. These substances contain bioactive compounds that have anti-diabetic properties, including the ability to lower blood glucose levels and improve insulin sensitivity. However, more research is needed to determine the optimal dose, duration, and safety of using bitter substances for managing diabetes. Patients with diabetes should consult with a healthcare provider before using bitter substances as a treatment for diabetes.

49. Can a diabetic patient undergo a surgery?

Yes, a diabetic patient can undergo surgery, but it requires careful planning and management. Poorly managed diabetes can increase the risk of complications during and after surgery. However, with proper preoperative preparation, intraoperative care, and postoperative management, the risk can be minimized, and the surgery can be performed safely.

Preoperative preparation:

Before the surgery, the patient's blood glucose levels must be under control to minimize the risk of complications. This can be achieved through proper medication management, dietary changes, and exercise. The patient may need to adjust their diabetes medications or insulin doses before the surgery. The healthcare team will also evaluate the patient's overall health and assess for any underlying conditions that may affect the surgery's safety.

Intraoperative care:

During the surgery, the healthcare team must monitor the patient's blood glucose levels carefully. An anesthesiologist will administer anesthesia and manage the patient's vital signs during the surgery. The surgeon will perform the surgery while working closely with the anesthesiologist and the rest of the healthcare team. The length of the surgery and the type of procedure can affect the patient's blood glucose levels, and the team will monitor and adjust the insulin and glucose levels as needed.

Postoperative management:

After the surgery, the patient may need to stay in the hospital for a few days to recover. The healthcare team will continue to monitor the patient's blood glucose levels and provide appropriate diabetes management. The patient may need to adjust their medications or insulin doses after the surgery. The healthcare team will also monitor for any complications, such as infections, delayed wound healing, or nerve damage.

Overall, the risks of surgery in diabetic patients depend on several factors, such as the patient's age, overall health, and the type and length of the surgery. Diabetic patients may be at higher risk for complications such as infection, delayed wound healing, or heart and kidney problems.

However, with proper preoperative preparation, intraoperative care, and postoperative management, the risk can be minimized.

It is essential for the diabetic patient to communicate openly with their healthcare team about their diabetes management and any concerns they may have about the surgery. The healthcare team will work together to create a personalized plan that meets the patient's unique needs and ensures a safe and successful surgery.

In summary, diabetic patients can undergo surgery with careful planning and management. It is crucial for the patient to work closely with their healthcare team to ensure their diabetes is well-controlled before, during, and after the surgery. The healthcare team will monitor the patient's blood glucose levels and provide appropriate diabetes management to minimize the risk of complications. With proper care and management, diabetic patients can undergo surgery safely and successfully.

50. What is the best way to reduce the blood sugar level in the morning before eating breakfast?

Maintaining healthy blood sugar levels is important for overall health and can help prevent diabetes and other health problems. If you find that your blood sugar levels are elevated in the morning, there are several things you can do to bring them down. Here are some tips based on verified information and realistic approaches:

Get regular exercise: Exercise helps improve insulin sensitivity, allowing your body to better use the insulin it produces to regulate blood sugar levels. This can help lower your blood sugar levels in the morning. Aim for at least 30 minutes of moderate exercise most days of the week.

Eat a balanced breakfast: Skipping breakfast can cause your blood sugar levels to spike later in the morning. Eating a breakfast that includes protein, healthy fats, and complex carbohydrates can help stabilize your blood sugar levels. Examples of balanced breakfasts include eggs with whole-grain toast and avocado, oatmeal with nuts and berries, or a vegetable omelet.

Limit high-carbohydrate foods: Foods that are high in carbohydrates, particularly simple sugars, can cause your blood sugar levels to spike. Avoiding sugary cereals, pastries, and juices can help prevent this. Instead, choose foods that are high in fiber and complex carbohydrates, such as whole-grain bread, fruits, and vegetables.

Get enough sleep: Lack of sleep can increase insulin resistance, which can lead to higher blood sugar levels. Aim for 7-8 hours of sleep per night to help keep your blood sugar levels in check.

Monitor your medication: If you take medication to manage your blood sugar levels, it's important to follow your doctor's instructions carefully. Take your medication as prescribed and monitor your blood sugar levels regularly. If you notice that your levels are consistently high in the morning, talk to your doctor about adjusting your medication.

Drink water: Drinking water can help flush out excess glucose from your bloodstream and help lower your blood sugar levels. Aim to drink at least 8 glasses of water per day.

Manage stress: Stress can cause your body to release hormones that raise your blood sugar levels. Finding ways to manage stress, such as practicing meditation, deep breathing, or yoga, can help keep your blood sugar levels in check.

In conclusion, there are several things you can do to help lower your blood sugar levels in the morning before eating breakfast. These include getting regular exercise, eating a balanced breakfast, limiting high-carbohydrate foods, getting enough sleep, monitoring your medication, drinking water, and managing stress. By making these lifestyle changes, you can help prevent diabetes and other health problems and improve your overall health and wellbeing.

Here are 30 facts about Diabetes you need to know.

1. Diabetes is a chronic medical condition characterized by high blood sugar levels.

2. There are two main types of Diabetes: Type 1 and Type 2.

3. Type 1 Diabetes is an autoimmune disease that occurs when the immune system attacks and destroys the cells in the pancreas that produce insulin.

4. Insulin is a hormone that regulates blood sugar levels.

5. Type 1 Diabetes is typically diagnosed in children and young adults, but it can occur at any age.

6. Type 2 Diabetes is the most common form of Diabetes and occurs when the body becomes resistant to insulin or does not produce enough insulin to regulate blood sugar levels.

7. Type 2 Diabetes is often linked to obesity, physical inactivity, and poor diet.

8. Gestational Diabetes is a form of Diabetes that occurs during pregnancy and usually resolves after delivery.

9. Diabetes can cause a range of complications, including kidney disease, nerve damage, vision problems, and cardiovascular disease.

10. Diabetes is the seventh leading cause of death worldwide.

11. In 2019, an estimated 463 million adults had Diabetes, representing 9.3% of the global adult population.

12. The number of people with Diabetes is expected to rise to 700 million by 2045.

13. Diabetes is more prevalent in low- and middle-income countries than in high-income countries.

14. Diabetes is often undiagnosed, particularly in low- and middle-income countries.

15. Diabetes is a major risk factor for heart disease and stroke.

16. People with Diabetes are two to four times more likely to die from heart disease than people without Diabetes.

17. Diabetes is the leading cause of kidney failure.

18. Diabetes is the leading cause of blindness in adults.

19. Diabetes is the leading cause of non-traumatic amputations.

20. Diabetes can also cause erectile dysfunction in men.

21. Diabetes can cause neuropathy, which is nerve damage that can result in numbness, tingling, and pain in the hands and feet.

22. Diabetes can cause gastroparesis, a condition in which the stomach takes too long to empty its contents.

23. Diabetes can cause hypoglycemia, or low blood sugar, which can be life-threatening if not treated promptly.

24. People with Diabetes need to monitor their blood sugar levels regularly.

25. Treatment for Diabetes typically involves lifestyle changes, such as healthy eating and exercise, as well as medication and insulin therapy.

26. Diabetes can often be prevented or delayed through lifestyle changes, such as maintaining a healthy weight, getting regular exercise, and eating a balanced diet.

27. There is currently no cure for Diabetes.

28. Research is ongoing to find new treatments and potential cures for Diabetes.

29. Diabetes research is funded by government agencies, foundations, and private organizations.

30. The cost of Diabetes care and treatment is a significant economic burden on individuals and healthcare systems worldwide.

Dr. Chri Allan wishes you Good Health!

....

Good Job on the completion of this book!

Knowledge is Power!

Now that you are aware, you are out of the trap of fear!

You may want to read any of my other books

HEALTHY HABITS FOR MEN!

HEALTHY HABITS FOR WOMEN!

NOTIFICATION FATIGUE!

PSORIASIS FACTS

KNOW THE FACS ABOUT CANCER

Check them out!